Visualizing and Verbalizing

For Language Comprehension and Thinking

Nanci Bell

REVISED EDITION

ISBN 0-945-856-01-6

Dedication

This book is dedicated to all my children

To Rody
for his warmth, wit, and intelligence

To Alison
for her wholeness, friendship, and spirit
and

To Rhett
who lives in my heart and is ever with me

Acknowledgements

I want to acknowledge the following friends and associates for their continuing contribution to this work: Phyllis Lindamood, Paul Worthington, Rody Bell, Kim Tuley, David Conway, Cathy Silva, Wendy Erb, Diane Budden, Pat Lamouria, Peg Klotz, Mike Franklin, Walter Conway, Julie Conway, Tim Conway, Callie Main, Betty Winholtz, Chuck Dyer, Melody Rulison, Vickie Blackman, Olive Swenson, Kathy Arnette, Anita Williams, Gayle Moyers, Stephen McCrocklin, Claudia Chervenak, Tina Semonsen, Chesterlyn Becerra, Marna Scarry-Larkin, Nina Moore, Trish Peake, Lisa Serrano, Chris Carlson, Polly Ralph, Ellen Lathrop, Jan Scarbrough, Shonna Grady, and Pam Mauro.

I especially want to acknowledge two very important women in my life who contributed in different ways to who I am:

> *My mother, Marietta Taylor, for her sparkle, sense of humor, pragmatism, courage, little-red-hen-attitude, and ability to humble me! After proudly giving her the first copy of my book, waiting and waiting for her to read it, and finally asking her if she had read it yet—she looked at me and said, "Did you have to make it so long?!" I miss her.*

> *My friend and long-time associate, Pat Lindamood, for her belief in me as a person of gift, her incredible patience with life, and her "We'll just keep on keeping on Nanci, dear" attitude. I'm not ready to miss her yet.*

Forward

I write the foreword for this work on *Visualizing and Verbalizing for Language Comprehension* with great pleasure, and yet with great concern. Will my words convey what a very significant contribution to the field of education and to teachers' and students' needs is within these pages? These concepts will change lives in profound ways, and both teachers and students will experience this impact.

If the sequence for imagery stimulation presented in the following pages is followed, it produces remarkable results. Individuals become able to visualize and comprehend language whose previous language processing could best be described as "in one ear and out the other." They also become able to organize and relevantly choose and order what they want to say, rather than giving so few or so many unorganized details that the message is garbled. Faces that have been passive and blank become animated. Hands and bodies that have been somehow separated from language become a part of it, actively participating and helping to create the visual images that make words come alive.

I have first-hand knowledge of these wonderful changes that are possible. I have not exaggerated. It may sound like magic, but it is not. It involves intense work with directed questions that focus on the students' responses; probing for what is there and what isn't there, so nothing is assumed; so that words are turned into richly detailed sensory images that are experienced vicariously but nonetheless personally.

For more than sixteen years I have had a close personal and professional association with Nanci Bell. In a clinical practice in speech-language and learning disabilities, and also in instructing university courses for teachers and other professionals, I have seen Nanci's sensitive spirit and inquiring and creative mind rise to the challenge of helping other minds strive toward their potential. Nanci has captured her charisma as well as her techniques in these pages. Those who make an effort to make them their own will enter into a more productive, more exciting experience with language than they have previously known. Teachers' joy in teaching will only be matched by their students' joy in finding the way into the PROCESS of learning. Thinking and communicating will become available to many through these visualizing/verbalizing concepts.

There is a striking parallel between the work my husband and I are doing in auditory conceptual judgment and its relationship to literacy skills and this work in visualizing and its relationship to spoken and written language comprehension. In both areas, educators have assumed a base of function which does not exist for many individuals until it is directly stimulated and developed.

Auditory conceptual judgment enables us to compare the identity and order of sounds in words. It provides a base for *thinking* about how to pronounce words, and how to spell and read them. Visualizing/verbalizing involves comparing the identity and order of words in phrases and sentences through the images they present. Comparing the images helps us to order and comprehend the information and concepts presented by words.

The new techniques offered in these two areas through our work and Nanci Bell's work are consistently effective in meeting sensory and language processing and integration problems previously unrecognized and unmet. These new more basic techniques fill gaps in traditional teaching procedures for phonics and word attack skills, and for reading comprehension, respectively. The gaps have existed because of erroneous assumptions about both students' and teachers' sound-sequencing and imagery abilities on the part of those who prepare materials for teachers.

It has been assumed that everyone can think accurately about sounds and their order in words, if one just pays attention and tries. It has also been assumed that everyone can create images for words. When poor performance is evident, and interestingly, significant numbers of teachers as well as students do not process easily and well in these two areas, the blame is often placed on lack of motivation or lower intellectual ability. The reality is that both areas of processing involve sensory information and language connections, and a sequence of intervention procedures appears to be necessary for significant numbers of individuals before they have access to auditory conceptual judgment for self-correction in speech, spelling, and reading, and visual imagery for language comprehension.

The concept of identifying sounds and their order in words is not new. Nor is the concept of visual imagery new. What is new in the Lindamood work in auditory conceptual judgment and Nanci Bell's work in visualizing/verbalizing is that NOTHING IS ASSUMED. A sequence of procedures so basic is offered in both areas that 1) the processing is accelerated and further refined for those who can access it readily; and 2) the emergence and development of the processing is stimulated for those who otherwise don't develop it.

Patricia Lindamood
November 1986

Preface

This book is written for two reasons: to **identify** and **solve** a problem. The content is very specific.

Gestalt imagery is a primary factor basic to the process involved in oral and written language comprehension, language expression, and critical thinking. It is the sensory information that connects us to language and thought. However, many individuals—both children and adults—have weakness in creating mental images and thereby have weak reading comprehension, weak oral language comprehension, weak verbal skills, and poor critical thinking.

This book identifies the importance of the sensory connection that imagery provides and teaches specific techniques for cognitive development and cognitive retraining. The steps stimulate auditory comprehension, reading comprehension, verbal expression, and higher order thinking skills—reasoning.

It is my hope that the pages of this book will make a contribution to the field of education and the lives of individuals. This is not about a learning style or a learning tool. This is about learning.

Nanci Netto Bell
May, 1991

Contents

Part One—The Concept

Part Two—The Process

Part Three—The Summary

The Concept

If I can't picture it,
I can't understand it.

Albert Einstein

Chapter 1

"I make movies when I read"

As I sit at this keyboard, sighing with fatigue, feet cold, and resentment building that I'm not back in bed, I wonder where to begin. My mind scans many options but settles on the puzzle of Catherine.

Catherine was an attractive high school senior who was brought to me for a learning disability evaluation. She could recognize words at a high school level, she could spell at a high school level, and she could read in context at a twelfth grade level with only three errors on the adult level paragraph. Her word attack skills were at the top of the test norm and her oral vocabulary was within normal range for her age level.

Here was a 17 year-old girl who could read adult level material, could spell adequately, had a sufficient oral vocabulary, but also had a problem. *She was failing nearly all her classes and would not graduate with her class.* She was flunking out of high school. Her parents and teachers were convinced that she had a "motivation" problem and/or an "attitude" problem. They didn't know what else might be wrong with her.

What was wrong with Catherine is also wrong with many other children and adults. Catherine had a language comprehension dysfunction. *She could read at a twelfth grade level but her comprehension was unstable after the third grade paragraph.* Her reading rate was good, with few decoding errors, but she had little idea of content. She could not recall nor interpret information from short paragraphs. Her oral reading comprehension was at the *9th percentile* and her silent reading comprehension was at the *10th percentile.* Since the 50th percentile indicates average performance, these scores were very low and placed her significantly below the performance level for other students at her age and grade level.

Catherine had been in school for 12 years. She had nine months of second grade, nine months of third grade, nine months of fourth grade, nine months of fifth grade, nine months of sixth grade, and so on through twelfth grade. The year-end tests had indicated weak reading comprehension since third grade. But, her reading comprehension had never developed.

Catherine could not remember what she read in even short paragraphs. What did she do to study for a test in science or history, where she had *chapters* to read and recall? She told me, *"I read things three and four times to get it...and then sometimes I still don't understand it.* It takes me a very long time to study...and when I do, I still fail the tests...so I have just given up."

She could read the words fine and she understood the meaning of each individual word, but when they all went together and formed concepts—she couldn't connect the information and comprehend. She didn't fit in a special reading class because she could "read." And, although her comprehension was weak, no one knew what to do about it—other than have her read and answer questions.

What was *causing* Catherine's problem? Why couldn't she remember what she read? What is the brain process that enables us to comprehend?

As I think about the above questions, my mind races back through the years to how this all began and a specific day and specific events that led to an answer. I recall a small office, just big enough to fit a small desk and three chairs. A wall phone is behind me, a two-drawer file cabinet, and a bookshelf. It is a room in a medical clinic and medical scenes are happening everywhere in the building, except in my little office. Here people learn to read and spell.

As I walk toward my office, I experience the pediatric wing of the medical clinic. Children crying, babies wrapped in blankets, parents reading books to scared little faces, and a busy, colorful fish tank. My office is past the waiting room, down the hall, and across from an optimistic, outspoken pediatrician and his examining rooms. As I walk into my office, I am within 10 steps of the end of the room. There is enough space for a window, the small desk, a phone, filing cabinet, and the three chairs.

It is late in the afternoon. I am sagging in the chair but semi-hovering over my student with the last remnants of my intensity. He is a college student, named Allen, majoring in architecture, and here to remediate a spelling dysfunction. We are developing his auditory conceptualization for sounds within words and are applying this to the multisyllable level of reading and spelling. We need a break in the spelling lesson so I ask him to read some material to me and give a verbal summary.

I hand Allen the skill book and have him read aloud to be sure he is decoding accurately. When he completes the page, I take the book and ask him to summarize what he has read.

His summary is incredible. He starts with the main idea and then proceeds to give me details. He infers, concludes, predicts, and evaluates the material. He seems enraptured, or at least involved, in the content.

As I think back to that time, I see myself staring at him. Truly astonished, I say, "That was really an incredible summary. How were you able to do that?"

His surprised reply is, "I don't know." Then, after some prodding, he adds, "**I just make movies when I read.**" I am staring at him. What a simple statement...I make movies when I read. He continues, with curiosity, "Don't you?"

"Don't I what? Make movies when I read?" I have to stop and think. Collecting myself, I ask in a professional voice, "What do you mean you make movies when you read?"

Allen replies, "I just see movies inside my head when I read. The words turn into pictures and I just remember the pictures. Doesn't that happen for everyone? Don't you see movies when you read?"

Very professional, "Yes, I guess I do. I just never thought about it. I don't know if everyone or anyone else does."

We discuss this phenomenon a little more and then Allen heads down the hall, dodging and stepping over the little people waiting to see the doctor.

Left alone in my office, I sit back and try to think about what seems to be a singularly important session. Do I visualize as I read? Thinking about *Gone with the Wind*, I can definitely say that I visualized those pages of southern life. Scarlet, Rhett Butler, the Civil War...all returned to me in the form of images.

Questions race through my mind. Do I visualize when I think and remember, as well as when I read? Does everybody visualize? Allen has the most complete comprehension I have ever seen, but what about students with weak comprehension. Do they visualize?

A few more weeks pass and another session seems to shed more light on this question. An Asian gentleman comes to me with a severe reading problem. He had a stroke five years earlier and has had a number of years of speech therapy that have successfully enabled him to regain his articulation. However, he is now experiencing much difficulty organizing his thoughts and expressing himself verbally. He tries to explain to me what is bothering him. He owns a chain of stores locally, and he is very concerned that he can't remember what he reads or what people say to him. He is relegated to menial tasks such as stocking shelves in his own store. He continues to try to explain to me that he can't remember what he reads or what he hears. He begins to gesture with his hands as he tries to say that "Words go in one ear and out the other." He is telling me that he has no way to keep the thoughts in his head...and it is very frustrating for him. He can't connect to language, either written language or oral language.

I recall Allen, the college student. He has "movies" of those words—concepts—as they come into his head. He visualized automatically, without effort. Can it be that this gentleman doesn't connect to the words because he doesn't visualize easily?

I have the Asian man read a primary-level paragraph, consisting of three very simple sentences. He reads the words adequately but he doesn't know what the story is about. I ask him, "Did you imagine—visualize—anything as you read the story? Did the words change into pictures in your head?"

After considerable thought, he replies, "No."

I ask again, just to be sure. "Are you sure? Did you use your imagination as you read? Did you picture anything in your mind when you read?"

He replied, "I saw nothing...there is nothing."

I ask a few questions regarding the story content, but he is unable to recall any information and is becoming embarrassed. I'd better check another way. This time I read a story to him. Nothing is imagined and very little is retained. After probing, he finally tells me one small detail. "The story was about an animal...I think." He doesn't image and he doesn't comprehend.

Those events were years ago and they directly led to an answer concerning reading comprehension and thinking. I pursued the concept initiated by Allen's casual statement, "I make movies in my head." I asked my students, children and adults, if they made images in their head when they read. Did they visualize? I got two types of responses: "Yes" from those students with good comprehension and "No" from those students with weak comprehension. When I asked the latter group to really stop and consider my question, their responses ranged from "Heaven's no"... "Of course not"... "What do you mean *see* something?"... "No, should I?"... to... "No, and I can't remember what I read."

Now, after much experience and research, it is my premise that visualizing is an answer as to *how* we process language and thought. *The brain "sees" in order to store and process information.* Both thinking and language comprehension are founded in imagery. Individuals with good language comprehension visualize concepts and form imaged gestalts. Individuals with weak language comprehension do not visualize concepts and therefore don't easily connect to language.

- Is visualizing related to language comprehension? *Yes.*
- And thinking? *Yes.*
- Is this what was causing Catherine's problem? *Yes.*

Visualization is directly related to language comprehension, language expression, and critical thinking. Imagery is a primary sensory connection in the brain.

Chapter 2

Gestalt Imaging and Cognition

L anguage comprehension is the ability to connect to and interpret both oral and written language. It is the ability to recall facts, get the main idea, make an inference, draw a conclusion, predict/extend, and evaluate. It is the ability to reason from language that is heard and language that is read. It is cognition.

Unfortunately, my clinical research and experience with Catherine—and many others like her—suggests the existence of a specific *Language Comprehension Disorder*. Bell (1991), "This comprehension disorder underlies the reading process and goes beyond use of context, phonological processing, word recognition, vocabulary, prior knowledge, and background experience...It is a disorder in the comprehension of both oral and written language and is based in the sensory system. It is a weakness in creating a gestalt." Gestalt is defined as a complex organized unit or whole that is more than the sum of its parts. The whole may have attributes that require a certain function for each part in the whole; these attributes are not deducible from analysis of the parts in isolation. In the case of a language comprehension disorder, the weakness in creating an imaged gestalt—whole— interferes with the *connection to* and *interpretation* of incoming language.

For many individuals, gestalts are not easily or successfully processed. Instead, "parts," bits and pieces, facts and details, dates and names are processed but not the entirety of the concept. Catherine's phenomenon was described as, "the words go in one ear and out the other." A high school student commented on his reading as, "It is words man...just words." A university graduate described listening to a lecture as, "It is like the language was written on a blackboard and someone was going behind and erasing it, and I only got parts"—not the gestalt.

However you believe it is created, the gestalt is the issue. The only reason to read or listen to language—take in verbal stimuli—is to get meaning, to comprehend, to interpret, to reason. And *the gestalt is a prerequisite to interpretation and reasoning*. For example, the main idea cannot be discerned if only a few "parts" have been grasped. An adequate inference cannot be determined or an accurate conclusion drawn from "parts." The gestalt is the entity from which the interpretive skills of identifying the main idea, inferring, concluding, predicting, extending, and evaluating can be processed. It enables the reader or listener to bring meaning to what is read or heard. It is an integral part of cognition.

If so critical, how does one create the gestalt? An answer: *imagery. Gestalt imagery is the ability to create an imaged whole.* **"Readers or listeners construct mental models of the situation a writer or speaker is describing. This is the basis of language comprehension"** Bower (1990). Kosslyn (1983), **"A number of great thinkers, most notably Albert Einstein, professed to rely heavily on imagery in their work.** Consider these words of Einstein: 'The psychical entities which seem to serve as elements of thought are certain signs and more or less clear *images* which can be "voluntarily" reproduced...this combinatory play seems to be the essential feature in productive thought—before there is any connection with logical construction of words or other kinds of signs which can be communicated to others.'

Imaging is a *sensory link* to language and thought. Gestalt imagery connects us to incoming language—both oral and written—and links us to and from prior knowledge, accesses background experiences, establishes vocabulary, and creates and stores information in both long term and short term memory. Vivid gestalt imaging may even be considered a "vicarious experience." Researchers in reading and imagery have produced direct evidence linking reading and mental imagery as well as studied the relationship of imagery to prior knowledge and thinking processes (Stemmler 1969; Richardson 1969; Paivio 1971,1986; Marks 1972; Sheehan 1972; Levin 1973, 1981; Pressley 1976; Sadoski 1983; Kosslyn 1983; Tierney & Cunningham 1984; Peters and Levin 1986).

Historical Perspective

There is considerable evidence in the field of both cognitive psychology and reading that supports imagery as a critical factor in language comprehension. Thus, before proceeding further, we'll examine some historical perspective regarding the relationship between imagery and cognition.

In all the research I compiled and all the articles I read, the most interesting was Aristotle in 348 B.C. In "On Memory and Recollection" he wrote, *"It is impossible even to think without a mental picture. "* In summarizing the section on memory, he continued, "Thus we have explained that memory or remembering is a state induced by mental images related as a likeness to that of which it is an image."

Simonides (556-468 B.C.) taught people to use imagery to improve their memories. His system was taught to many Greek and Roman orators, who without notes or cues cards, sometimes spoke for several hours. After I read Aristotle and Simonides I wondered what happened to the practice and art of imagery. I found that Simonides' memory system and Aristotle's theory of memory and recollection, both emphasizing the critical role of imagery, comprised the classical art of memory for over a thousand years. Then neo-Platonic ideas, modifications of Plato's ideas, began to gradually remove it from prominence. In the 11th and 12th centuries, memory systems again became useful for purposes of remembering and making memorable the central Christian ideas. Thomas Aquinas was largely responsible for the renewed interest in the classical techniques for stimulating memory and he wrote, *"Man's mind cannot understand thoughts without images of them."*

Although the relationship between imagery and memory was well understood in those early centuries, in post-Renaissance time imagery related to memory training declined. Perhaps the Protestant Reformation that disparaged the use of images in sculpture and arts, also diminished it in schools. Fortunately, since about the 1950's there has been renewed interest in imagery, and an increased interest in the last few years.

Moving to more contemporary times, Jean Piaget (1936, cited by Bleasdale 1983) wrote in favor of a perceptual base to memory. According to Piaget, knowledge structures, or schemata, are acquired when the infant actively manipulates, touches, and interacts with the environment. As objects are manipulated, sensory-motor schemata are developed and changed to accommodate new information. Over time, *schemata become internalized in the form of imaged thought.* Piaget further stated, "It is clear that imaginal representations are not formed with the same facility in each case, and that there is therefore a hierarchy of image levels, which may correspond to stages of development... *The evolution of images is a kind of intermediate between that of the perceptions and that of the intelligence."*

Proceeding chronologically, we'll examine some of the more interesting research and historical commentary. Arnheim (1966) wrote, "Thinking is concerned with the objects and events of the world we know... When the objects are not physically present, they are represented indirectly by what we remember and know about them. *In what shape do memory and knowledge deliver the needed facts? In the shape of memory images, we answer most simply. Experiences deposit images."* He quoted the psychologist Edward B. Titchener, '...my mind, in its ordinary operations, is a fairly complete picture gallery, not of finished paintings, but of impressionist notes. Whenever I read or hear that somebody has done something modestly, or gravely, or proudly, or humbly, or courteously, I see a visual hint of the modesty or pride or humility.' The *visual hint* may be a means of processing abstract material.

Continuing into the sixties, Allan Paivio (1969), who has written extensively on imagery and cognition, stated, "As every psychologist knows, imagery once played a prominent role in the interpretation of associative meaning, mediation, and memory. It was widely regarded as the mental representative of meaning—or of concrete meaning at least. William James, for example, suggested that *the static meaning of concrete words consists of sensory images awakened* [1890]."

The seventies brought further illumination from Paivio (1971). He had been attempting to demonstrate the way in which imagery can affect the acquisition, transformation, or retrieval of different classes of information. *His dual coding theory for cognition emerged, defining imagery (usually visual imagery) as one of two types of cognitive code. The other type is verbal code.* Paivio suggests that linguistic competence and linguistic performance are based on a substrate of imagery. Imagery includes not only static representations of objects, but also dynamic representations of action sequences and relationships between objects and events.

Pribram (1971) stated, "Recently the importance of the Image concept has started to be recognized: cognitive psychologists analyzing the process of verbal learning have been faced with a variety of Imaging processes which demand neurological underpinnings... Neurological research as well as insights derived from the information-processing sciences, have helped make understandable the machinery which gives rise to this elusive ghost-making process." He further hypothesized that *"all thinking has, in addition to sign and symbol manipulation, a holographic component."*

Also in the seventies, Kosslyn (1976) conducted a developmental study on the effects and role of imagery in retrieving information from long-term memory. In two blocks of trials, first graders, fourth graders and adults were asked to determine whether or not various animals are characterized by various properties, first upon the consultation of a visual image and then without imagery. He reported that *imagery provided the most opportunity for retrieval.*

Related research came from Wepman's (1976) studies on aphasia. Aphasia is described as any partial or total loss of the faculty to articulate or understand speech, usually due to a brain lesion. Wepman observed dramatic improvement in expressive language when he stimulated the "embellishment" of thought through images. He approached aphasia and aphasia therapy from the viewpoint that the disorder was one of impairment of thought processing and that therapy should therefore concentrate on embellishment of receptive language. He reported that he had never seen such dramatic results prior to using imagery. This study indicated that imaging was critical to actual thought process which is compatible with my clinical experience. Stimulating imagery develops expressive speech in "normal" individuals. Individuals using images from which to speak become more organized

16

in their expressive language. They are more concise and more able to monitor their language for relevancy and sequential/logical thought expression.

There are other interesting writings in the seventies. Paul Pietsch (1975) speculated a global approach to memory, which treats memory as a phenomenon of the total brain. In 1965, two physicists, Bela Julesz and K.A. Pennington, proposed a similarity between the optical hologram and memory stored in the brain. Optical holograms reconstruct vividly realistic images. Although Pietsch attempted to dispute what Julesz and Pennington suggested, their theory survived every test and Pietsch concluded that memory is hologramatic and a process of the whole brain.

The eighties gave us additional evidence when Wittrock (1981) stated, "Reading comprehension is the generation of meaning for written language... We found that reading comprehension can be facilitated by several different procedures that emphasize attention to the text and to the construction of verbal or imaginal elaborations." In a study with fourth graders, compared with a control group of students given the same time to learn with the same reading teacher, he noted *"the generation of verbal and imaginal relations or associations between the text and experience increased comprehension approximately by fifty percent."*

Further research was conducted by Oliver (1982) with three experiments to determine if an instructional set for visual imagery would facilitate reading comprehension in elementary school children. He concluded, *"These findings indicate that teachers should try to help children develop the metacognitive skill of visual imagery as a strategy for improving comprehension... Visualization enhances comprehension."*

Sadoski (1984), in an abstract from a study with third and fourth graders, states, "Paivio (1983) and Sadoski (1983) have theorized that certain images evoked by stories and stored in memory can serve as 'conceptual pegs' for the storage and retrieval of story information...Anderson and Kulhavy (1972), Kulhavy and Swenson (1975), and Gambrell (1982) have found that *school-age readers instructed to image while reading recalled more and made significantly more predictive inferences about story events than did control group subjects."* The study supports the "contention that imagery can serve as a comprehension strategy, as a mental peg for memory storage, retrieval, and redintigration, and as a repository of deeper meanings that utilize text information."

Sadoski's inquiry continued. Sadoski, Goetz, Kangiser (1988) studied 39 college students. The students read "three short stories with similar plot structures and rated each story by paragraph according to one of three criteria: the degree of mental imagery evoked, the degree of emotion evoked, or the degree of importance to the story as a whole...The relationships found between imagery, affect and importance are related to current theories of basic psychological processes in reading." They concluded from the study that, *"The prediction that imagery in reading stories may serve as a unifying comprehension strategy and serve thematic purposes is consistent with the results of our earlier studies...* These findings also support Paivio's (1986) dual coding theory and his contention that there is a parallel, nonverbal dimension to discourse processing which can be analyzed, and which contributes to the overall comprehension, integration, and appreciation of text."

And, 1989 provided the research of Long, Winograd, and Bridge. They summarized their findings regarding imagery and reading: "Our results suggest that imagery may be involved in the reading process in a number of ways. First, imagery may increase the capacity of working memory during reading by assimilating details and propositions into chunks which are carried along during reading. Second, imagery seems to be involved in making comparisons or analogies—that is, in matching schematic and textual information. Third, *imagery seems to function as an organizational tool for coding and storing meaning gained from the reading.*"

Into the nineties, Sadoski, Goetz, Olivarez Jr., Lee, and Roberts (1990) investigated "the spontaneous use of imagery and its relationship to free verbal recall with Community college students, who read a 2,100-word story under one of three sets of instructions and then recalled the story and reported their images immediately and 48 hours later... *Images of the story were much more prevalent in memory two days later than verbal recall, further suggesting a distinction in processes and the power of imagery in reading a story...* This study contributes to a series of studies that suggest that imagery is a distinctive aspect of reading viable for study in its own right... During the last twenty years, mental imagery has become a topic of increasing interest to cognitive researchers, to the extent that it is ' one of the hottest topics in cognitive science' (Block, 1981). Led by Paivio (1971, 1986), Shepard (1978), Kosslyn (1980), and others, the study of imagery in cognition has risen from the status of a secondary or 'epiphenomenal' mental process to one which rivals propositional network theories as a basis for cognition."

Clark and Paivio (1991) state, *"Dual Coding Theory (DCT) explains human behavior and experience in terms of dynamic associative processes that operate on a rich network of modality-specific verbal and nonverbal (or imagery) representations.* The research demonstrates that concreteness, *imagery*, and verbal associative processes play major roles in various educational domains: the representation and comprehension of knowledge, learning and memory of school material, effective instruction, individual differences, achievement motivation and test anxiety, and the learning of motor skills."

Symptoms of Gestalt Imagery Weakness

Although imagery has been viewed with prominence in learning theory, specifically Paivio's dual coding theory for cognition, two problems exist: the ability to image gestalts is often assumed in the educational arena and gestalt imagery does not appear to be readily available to many individuals. First, we must have assumed imagery processing, or we would have placed imagery in the curriculum to develop language comprehension in the classroom. Second, many individuals do have weak gestalt imagery that creates a commonality of symptoms, ranging from mild to severe. They often display a range of symptoms, with poor reading comprehension the most evident.

Reading Comprehension

For example, as we noted with Catherine, during and after reading (either aloud or silently), individuals experience only processing "parts" of what has been read. Thus, they often reread material numerous times in order to understand it. They experience difficulty accessing and integrating old information with new and although their vocabulary may be adequate for isolated words, they have difficulty bringing the words together to form imaged gestalts.

Anecdotal references often serve to clarify theory. Some additional individual cases, all of whom experienced difficulty imaging gestalts, will assist you in *"gestalting"* the symptoms of this disorder. A college graduate with good decoding and above average intelligence, attempting to enter medical school, described his reading comprehension disability as "not having a cognitive tool kit... I opened up my cognitive tool kit and there was something missing. Others seemed to do this (comprehend) very easily. I could never understand how they did it and why I couldn't... About 20% of what I took in stayed and about 80% went out or was just parts." Another college student, again with good vocabulary and good decoding, but on academic probation described, "There wasn't one thing I could do right. I didn't remember anything I read. It was very frustrating. I read each sentence three times and then went on to the next sentence and read it three times. It didn't make any sense put together...if I read the information enough times I could remember it for maybe 30 seconds and then I had no clue."

Many comprehension problems exist in our classrooms. Although we have been aware of the importance of comprehension, we have not known how to teach it. Reading teachers have been aware of the taxonomy of comprehension skills that need to be taught, such as main idea, inference, conclusions, prediction, and evaluation. However, they have not understood how to teach these skills. Commonly, the instructional procedures for developing comprehension are to simply have students read material and answer questions. Sometimes this means answering questions at the end of a chapter or going through a skill book and answering the questions after reading a short paragraph. However, *reading and answering questions is testing comprehension not teaching comprehension.*

Often children who read well but have weak comprehension are not placed in special reading classes. And, as stated above, even if they are placed in special classes, the remediation is too often just reading and answering questions. Unfortunately, without developing imagery to form gestalts, the child's comprehension skills usually remain weak, resulting in continued frustration and poor performance.

The following is an example of children with reading comprehension problems, who have now progressed to the twelfth grade. It is also an example of the effectiveness of Visualizing/Verbalizing which successfully develops imagery and comprehension.

> The superintendent of a small high school called the Lindamood Language and Literacy Center for assistance with students who were not passing the reading part of the proficiency test, which is necessary for high school graduation in California. Decoding weakness (difficulty reading words) was anticipated, but instead most of the students were able to read paragraphs through the tenth and twelfth grades with very few decoding errors. Their problem was that they could not recall information at that level. After all those years of school, most students still had to be taken as far back as the third and fourth grade passages to get full recall. A senior boy explained, "It's just words, man." After two months of Visualizing/Verbalizing treatment, all but two of the students passed the proficiency test. Most of the students had less than 30 hours of treatment and of the eighteen students, only two students didn't pass—one had a severe decoding problem and the other minimal attendance. The same senior boy commented that he now read books for book reports rather than going to the movie. He said, *"Now, I turn the movies on in my head when I read. It's like being my own director."*

Reading comprehension requires *automatic* imaging in which parts are visualized and automatically brought together in the form of more images in order to develop a whole (gestalt) of the information read. Individuals without this ability will have a reading comprehension dysfunction that cannot be corrected by just reading more material and answering questions.

Oral Language Comprehension and Expression
Another common symptom is *weak oral language comprehension*. The same "parts to whole" problem exists. Individuals connect to parts in a conversation, parts in a lecture, parts in a movie, and parts in their thinking processes. They have difficulty responding relevantly and thinking logically. They often ask and reask the same question and may be labeled as poor listeners or inattentive. A teacher described that she always sat in the front row in a college class or at a professional conference in order to "try and keep the information from going past me." A husband complained because his wife, who was a college graduate, asked and reasked the same question. Unaware of her repetition, she simply rephrased the

same question a little differently each time. He explained that she didn't grasp the essence of his answer nor conversation in general.

The following are some symptoms of difficulty in processing oral language:

1. *Individuals may frequently not understand jokes.* Language humor depends on imagery, whereas sight humor (pie in face) does not and is more easily understood. Almost everyone gets sight gags but not everyone gets language-based humor.
2. *Individuals may not understand concepts of cause and effect.* To process cause and effect relationships you must be able to process a gestalt from which to judge an effect.
3. *Individuals may not respond to explanations given in language.* If a student's performance needs correcting, a "talking to" may be only partially understood or not understood at all, because the student is connecting to only a part of the oral explanation.
4. *Individuals may ask and reask questions that have already been answered.* The individual hears the answer but is unable to process and connect to the given information and will therefore ask the same question again, only phrased differently. Such individuals are often not aware that they are asking the same question over and over, only with modified language.
5. *Individuals may not grasp the main idea or inferences from television shows or movies, although they may get a few details.* The individual may seem to miss concepts or nuances from movies they've seen. In discussions with them they don't interpret the movie or story sequence well.
6. *Individuals may lose attention quickly in conversation or lectures.* Students who are unable to connect to the gestalt of language will find that in a few minutes, often less, they are "lost" and may drift away mentally and/or physically.
7. *Individuals may have weakness in auditory memory and following directions.*

These symptoms may be severe and labeled as aphasia. However, these may also be subtle weaknesses that cause others to suspect lack of intelligence or lack or motivation. In fact, frequently individuals with these symptoms will doubt their intelligence.

The oral language comprehension weakness is often accompanied by an *oral language expression weakness.* Individuals experience difficulty organizing their verbalization, expressing themselves easily and fluently, or they are verbal but scattered, relating information out of sequence. For example, a student on academic probation, with severely impaired auditory and reading comprehension, frequently interjected irrelevant comments in conversation. His comments were disjointed both unto themselves and to the topic. Consequently, he was often viewed as mentally disabled. After gestalt imagery stimulation—Visualizing and

Verbalizing—was nearly completed, he explained that previously he had desperately wanted to participate in conversation but was only able to comment on the "parts" he was able to grasp. So, he blurted out irrelevant comments.

The early days of developing the Visualizing/Verbalizing process resulted in my awareness of this symbiotic relationship between gestalt imagery and expressive oral language. For example, although the sessions were focused on stimulating visualization, expressive language was remarkably influenced. Individuals began to verbalize better. Their language was more organized, more descriptive, more relevant, and more fluent.

Expressive language weakness has two primary symptoms:

1. *Individuals may be described as "quiet" and unable to express themselves well.* Their gesturing while speaking may be limited and they seem generally uncomfortable with verbal expression. If severe enough, they may be labeled aphasic.

2. *Individuals may be verbal, but their verbalization is scattered and difficult to follow.* They may be "talkers" but their language isn't succinct and often loses focus because their thoughts lose focus. They are often described as *air-heads*.

Expressive language weakness, mild or moderate, contributes to problems in an individual's life. The person will have communication problems and may even be viewed as lacking intelligence. The following list is from a note to me from a mother regarding her sixth grade son, and the problems he experienced at home and in school. It aptly describes some of the symptoms of this dysfunction.

1. Memory and comprehension instability
2. Poor, slow, fatiguing reading ability
3. Messy handwriting/avoidance of written assignments
4. Bores easily
5. Can't do word problems in math
6. Can't express himself well
7. Seems to miss the main idea—only gets parts of what I say or he reads
8. Poor logical thinking, problem solving, and problem analysis
9. Difficulty following directions
10. Accused of daydreaming or being "spaced out" in classroom

Influence on Behavior
This language weakness seems to generate a range of symptoms. Individuals may exhibit poor auditory memory, difficulty following directions, or behavior problems. Although not all behavior problems can be attributed to language comprehension weakness, it is a factor to consider in many cases. Individuals who cannot grasp or

create gestalts from language generally have difficulty with the concept of "cause and effect." If they are connecting to parts, they are not able to comprehend the whole of a given situation. They may not appreciate the consequences of their actions and become frustrated with intervention that usually begins verbally. The "talking to" by parents or teachers may often be misunderstood or confused.

Also, classroom behavior may be influenced by weakness in language processing. Students with weakness in oral language comprehension may lose interest after a few sentences. They cannot attend to lectures, or the teacher, because within minutes they are lost. The language is not connecting and making sense, so they may begin to do other things to entertain themselves or they may just sit and appear to be "spaced out."

> I observed a teacher in a second-grade classroom present an art history lesson to his class. He was at the front of the room with his students seated on the rug in positions of choice. A number of children scurried to be in the first row, some chose the second row, while others chose the last row or scattered themselves a little farther from the front. As he presented the lesson, he was interesting, animated, and articulate for his second-grade learners. Initially all the students were attending and well behaved. They wanted to be "good." However, within a few minutes, some students began to lose attention, began wiggling, became moderately disruptive, and the teacher had to interrupt his presentation to bring them back to the lesson. What had happened?
>
> As I looked on, I wondered, "Are these behavior problems as they seem?" The lesson was presented orally. It was very probable that the students with inappropriate behavior had not been able to stay connected to the language. They initially attended to the lesson, but in only a few minutes were lost and disconnected. It is probable that their "behavior problems" were caused or contributed to by "language problems."

Weakness in Written Language Expression, Following Oral Directions, humor...
Weak written language expression is often another symptom. Though spelling and punctuation skills appear intact, writing may lack preciseness, organization, and specifics, and be described as several essays, rather than a coherent whole written to the topic. Additional symptoms include *difficulty following directions, difficulty judging cause and effect,* and a *weak sense of humor.* Unfortunately, the symptom of difficulty following oral directions is often diagnosed as Attention Deficit Disorder and medication subsequently prescribed.

Summary of Symptoms of Gestalt Imaging Weakness

• **Weak reading comprehension**

• **Weak oral language comprehension**

• **Weak oral language expression**

• **Weak written language expression**

• **Weak sense of humor**

• **Weakness in following directions**

• **Difficulty with "cause and effect"**

Causes and Contributors

This gestalt imagery—language comprehension—disorder is insidious in that it is often difficult to detect and effects the comprehension of both oral and written language. The causes are puzzling. Perhaps it is a hereditary factor, since usually one or both parents describe a similar deficiency. Perhaps a genetic basis for weak gestalt imagery will eventually be isolated. Perhaps with the advent of more sophisticated brain measurements a specific brain etiology will be determined. Perhaps comprehension has been assumed because the focus in the field of reading has been on decoding, and more recently on the context effect.

Or, perhaps a cause is lack of stimulation, an atrophying effect. Old-time radio and record stories created auditory stimuli that stimulated imagery. Currently, however, leisure time is spent engaging in a pastime that offers images rather than stimulates images. Television viewing not only provides images but also consumes what may have been reading time, storytelling time, and language interaction time—time that stimulated imagery.

Whatever the cause, gestalt imaging ability appears to be a separate function onto itself. *Although impaired phonological processing and decoding, weak oral vocabulary, and reduced prior knowledge and background of experiences may contribute to weak imaging during reading, these factors in and of themselves do not appear to be causal.* As stated earlier, many individuals with good vocabulary for isolated words *are not able* to comprehend written language efficiently. Also, many individuals with wide experiences and good educations *are not able* to comprehend efficiently. Many good decoders *are not able* to comprehend efficiently. In contrast, many poor decoders *are* able to comprehend efficiently. If concepts or content are presented to them orally, they appear brilliant in their ability to interpret and reason.

Although perhaps not causal, weak decoding can be a primary contributor to weak gestalt imagery during reading. An individual can have good imagery and good comprehension *only* if he or she can decode enough words critical to the integration and processing of the gestalt. A few decoding errors may cause ridiculous images, and necessitate rereading for contextual cues and correction. However, a severe phonological processing disorder, causing numerous decoding errors, may cause enough image distortion so as to interfere with comprehension.

Weak vocabulary also may interfere with gestalt imagery, if the unknown words are critical to the whole. If not critical to the gestalt, the imaged concept—context—may serve to stimulate vocabulary development. It is not clear which problem existed first—poor vocabulary or poor gestalt imagery—though it is evident that stimulating images for vocabulary aids in the storage and retrieval of meaning for isolated words. Smith, (1987), after a study with 142 university students, states, "The significant difference that occurred between the definition only and the definition and sentence and imagery groups supports Paivio's dual coding theory. In accord with Paivio's theory the visual image did provide an additional memory trace that improved long term memory for the vocabulary items in the study. This finding mirrors research spanning the years as far back as Kirkpatrick in 1894."

Prior knowledge and background experience also may interfere with comprehension and imaging. But, techniques to access prior knowledge such as first discussing material with children, first setting the scene, and first teaching vocabulary do not necessarily stimulate independent comprehension. The *individual* will need to set the scene by decoding, imaging, and interacting with stored images so as to have deep structure available for meaning. The individual will need to have imaging ability to hold and integrate vocabulary with incoming language and images—creating a gestalt.

Some Results After Stimulation of Gestalt Imagery/Comprehension

Clinical Data

It will be helpful at this point to examine some data after gestalt imagery/language comprehension stimulation. My energy has been in the area of clinical diagnosis and treatment, offered individually, to students of all ages. The primary focus of treatment is to develop either language comprehension or phonological processing, or a combination of both. This results in interesting individual case studies showing marked improvement in language processing. For example, the filling of the college graduate's cognitive tool kit. Before clinical treatment to develop concept imagery—language comprehension, he had twice taken the MCAT (Medical College Admissions Test) and received a score of four on the reading comprehension subtest. Since the average was eight, he said, "No medical schools will consider me." After ten weeks of intensive treatment, he was performing at the 98th percentile in reading comprehension. When he retook the MCAT he received a score of ten in reading comprehension, performing above average.

The following results are based on clinical study, thus there necessarily was no control group. At the Lindamood-Bell Learning Processes Center, forty-five individuals received clinical intervention—intensive therapy consisting of four hours of daily individual treatment—for whom the focus of treatment was *only* concept imagery—language comprehension stimulation. Each individual was diagnosed to determine receptive oral vocabulary, expressive oral vocabulary, phoneme segmentation ability, word attack, word recognition, oral reading paragraph comprehension, and silent reading comprehension. They ranged in age from nine to fifty-seven years old and included 22 males and 23 females: eighteen were in grades K-8; thirteen were in grades 9-12; five were in college; and nine were adults, primarily college graduates. Although performing poorly in reading comprehension, it is of interest to note their performance on other diagnostic tests. For example, 80% had age level-or-above receptive oral vocabulary skills and 71% had age level-or-above expressive oral vocabulary skills. Their performance on the Lindamood Auditory Conceptualization Test indicated that 88% had excellent phoneme segmentation ability. The Woodcock Word Attack Test indicated that 83% had above grade level word attack skills. The comprehension disorder clearly appeared to be isolated from the above factors.

Since energy has been given to each individual rather than to a group, each of the forty-five were not given the same pre and post tests. However, the following will report on the individuals that were given the same pre and post test from which statistical evidence can be evaluated. The average time in individual treatment was 47.26 hours, with a range from 16 to 110 hours.

Seventeen individuals, ranging in age from 11 to 57 years old were administered the Gray Oral Reading Test Revised. The percentile mean for the pre GORT-R Test was 43.94. The percentile mean for the post GORT-R Test was 75.55. This repeated measure showed highly significant effect for the group, p <.001.

Sixteen individuals ranging in age from 15 to 52 years old were administered the Descriptive Tests of Language Skills of the College Board, Reading Comprehension subtest. The percentile mean for the pre College Board was 56.06. The percentile mean for the post College Board was 71.29. Again, this repeated measure showed highly significant results for the group, p <.001.

Twenty-seven individuals, ranging in age from 11 to 59 years old, were administered the Detroit Tests of Learning Aptitude, Oral Directions subtest. The mental age level average for the pre Oral Directions subtest was 11.80 and the mental age level average for the post Oral Directions subtest was 14.33. The overall average gain in mental age was 2.53 years.

Chance Program

Motivation and interest can interfere with comprehension and active focus, but individuals with good comprehension appear to have access to automaticity in gestalt imaging. They appear to comprehend readily with ease. Their expenditure of energy is low because they function effortlessly. Many individuals with a Language Comprehension Disorder have been mislabeled lazy, not motivated, inattentive, and not interested. Graceland College in Iowa, a private liberal arts college, was considering a "motivation tract" for college students at risk, many on academic probation. In 1988 a study was conducted resulting in the Chance Program. Diagnostic testing indicated that a high percentage of students being considered for the motivation tract scored low on reading comprehension measurements. Thus a number of these students entered into a trial voluntary program, entitled the Chance Program, and were given direct stimulation to develop concept imagery, while continuing to attend their regular classes.

Diagnostic tests measuring oral vocabulary, phoneme segmentation, word attack, word recognition and paragraph comprehension were administered to the sixteen Chance Program students. The testing indicated good phoneme segmentation, good spelling, good word recognition, good word attack, low vocabulary, and poor reading comprehension. The mean beginning scores in vocabulary and reading comprehension were lower for the 16 students in the Chance Program as compared with a sample of 120 students, randomly selected from the student body. For example, in vocabulary and reading comprehension, the mean percentile ranking for the Chance Program students was 13.8 and 13.3, respectively. The mean percentile ranking in vocabulary and reading comprehension for the 120 students of the student body was 41.1 and 44.8, respectively.

After treatment to stimulate concept imagery, the Chance Program students demonstrated a significant gain in reading comprehension. On the Descriptive Tests of Language Skills of the College Board, Reading Comprehension subtest, the mean percentile ranking improved from the 29.8 percentile to the 51.6 percentile. On the Nelson-Denny Vocabulary the mean percentile ranking improved from the 13.8 percentile to the 22.1 percentile. On the Nelson-Denny Reading Comprehension the mean percentile ranking improved from the 13.3 percentile to the 33.1 percentile.

The gains made on the Nelson-Denny Comprehension Test were highly significant, $p < .001$. The gains made on the Nelson-Denny Vocabulary Test were significant, $p < .05$. The gains noted on the Descriptive Tests of Language Skills of the College Board, Reading Comprehension subtest, were also significant, $p < .05$.

Of further interest, the grade point average (G.P.A.) for the students' that received concept imagery treatment in the Chance Program improved from an average of 2.31 to 2.76. This is an eleven percent increase in G.P.A. and is more significant considering that fourteen of the sixteen students also had an increase in graded semester hours, from an average of 10.95 to 14.0. Because of the noted gains in comprehension and G.P.A., the status of the Chance program changed from a pilot study to inclusion in the curriculum at Graceland College.

Navajo Indian Reservation
An on-going Federal Projects study, Kimbrough (1991), at Window Rock Elementary School on the Navajo Indian Reservation studied the effects of the V/V Program on language comprehension with a sample population of fourth and fifth graders. The study represents the 1989-1990 school year, which is the first year of the project. The criteria for student selection was from the Iowa Tests of Basic Skills (ITBS), Reading Comprehension component. Students selected for remediation had a stanine score of 3 or below, (5 is average). The measured gains were based on National Curve Equivalent Scores (NCES) versus grade level equivalent scores. The project fourth and fifth graders received the Visualizing/Verbalizing Program thirty minutes/day for *five* weeks, in small groups. The overall average gain in reading comprehension was 6.6 points on the NCES. The national average gain is 3 points. Kimbrough states enthusiastically, "In the past, my students have always averaged a gain of 2 to 3 NCES points. After doing Visualizing/Verbalizing for 5 weeks preceding the ITBS testing in a remedial setting, my students far surpassed their level of the past."

The Right and Left Hemispheres

We ought not to leave this chapter without some discussion of hemispherisity and visualizing/verbalizing. That we have two hemispheres in our brain is by now widely written about and known. Most research indicates that the left side and right side of our brain are two semiautonomous systems that process information differently and can be used in a specialized manner.

It is believed the left brain is involved in logical, analytical, linear, sequential thought process and specific linguistic abilities. It controls the right side of the body. The right side of the brain is involved in spatial relations, musical, spiritual, intuitive, creative, and holistic thought processes. It controls the left side of the body.

Most research suggests that imagery is a function of the right hemisphere. "Internally visualizing requires the right cerebral hemisphere to dominate...The right hemisphere 'thinks' in images and the left hemisphere 'thinks' in words," Grayson H. Wheatly (1977).

"They are more alike than different—after all, they are nourished by the same food, go to the same parties, and face the same problems. But one seems specialized for dealing with things in sequences, the other for dealing with them all at once," Robert Ornstein (1978). He felt that, in essence, we have a whole brain with specialized parts; each of the hemispheres can process both sorts of material but it is not efficient to do so because they are similar in structure but different in function.

The hemispheres are specialized but related and most of the literature implies that imaging is a right hemisphere function. Perhaps it is, but I believe that there are at least *two* basic types of imaging. One type of imaging is *"concept imagery"* for thinking and comprehension. Concept imagery processes parts to a whole. This book is discussing concept—gestalt—imagery. The other type of imaging is *"symbol imagery"* for decoding and encoding letter symbols. Symbol imagery processes single letters and segments a whole into separate parts. Perhaps concept imagery is a right hemisphere function, and symbol imagery a left hemisphere function. The literature implies reading is in the left hemisphere. Or perhaps concept imagery is also in the left hemisphere, but a different part of the left hemisphere.

Whichever hemisphere, I am certain that concept and symbol imagery are not part of the same brain function. For example, many individuals can image for spelling letters but can't image concepts for comprehension and many individuals can image concepts for comprehension, which seems to be larger units, but can't see letters in their mind. Allen, the college student with excellent comprehension, had an auditory segmentation dysfunction and consequently a spelling dysfunction. He couldn't auditorily perceive sounds in words and he also couldn't visualize the letters associated with those sounds. I once asked him to visualize the letters in the word "cat" and he simply couldn't see them in his head. He could picture a fat cat, a white cat, a spotted cat, a cat on a red chair, but he just couldn't picture the letters "c-a-t."

Perhaps it is as simple as developing the interaction between both hemispheres. "Integration of the function of the two hemispheres is our real goal," Robert Samples (1975). Or as Konicek (1975) said, "When two living forces are combined, the end result is more than the sum of the parts." Stimulating one hemisphere will not weaken the other hemisphere, it will just enhance the integration and develop more complete processing.

Jerre Levy (1985) also reported that, after a whole career of studying how the two hemispheres relate to each other and to behavior, she is convinced that "we have a single brain that generates a single mental self." She quoted 17th century philosopher, Rene Descartes, who believed the brain must act as a unified whole in order to yield a unified mental world.

Levy continued with speculation about reading and brain activity, which supports the visualizing/verbalizing premise of this book. "When a person reads a story, the right hemisphere may play a special role in decoding visual information, maintaining an integrated story structure, appreciating humor and emotional content, deriving meaning from past associations and understanding metaphor. At the same time, the left hemisphere plays a special role in understanding syntax, translating written words into their phonetic representations and deriving meaning from complex relations among word concepts and syntax."

The Visualizing and Verbalizing (V/V) process that had been exploratory now also appears to be compatible in scope to the dual coding theory. Paivio (1971), "The most general assumption in dual coding theory is that there are two classes of phenomena handled cognitively by separate subsystems, one specialized for the representation and processing of information concerning nonverbal objects and events, the other specialized for dealing with language." Paivio (1986) said, **"The dual coding interpretation is straightforward. The concrete descriptive tasks require a high degree of referential exchange between the verbal and imagery systems."**

Levy's premise, and Paivio's dual coding theory, directly support the concept and treatment techniques of *Visualizing and Verbalizing*. The *visualization* (imagery) stimulation may activate one critical aspect of cognition (perhaps in the right cerebral hemisphere) and *verbalization* (semantic coding) stimulation may activate the other critical aspect of cognition (perhaps in the left cerebral hemisphere). Thus, stimulating an integration of brain activity.

Visualizing and Verbalizing was named from a *technique* that worked. It is encouraging that the technique now seems founded in theory.

Part Two

The Process

Now I turn the movies on in my head when I read.
It's like being my own director.

Anonymous
A young man in high school

Visualizing/Verbalizing Overview

The *Visualizing/Verbalizing* (V/V) process is very powerful. Once developed, it enables the individual to: 1) image parts and gestalts from oral and written language, 2) recall and relate the imaged gestalts, and 3) reorganize and verbalize concepts, using the imaged gestalt as a reasoning foundation. This results in significant improvement in:

1. *Reading Comprehension*
   Visualizing/Verbalizing enables the student to read material and comprehend it with more than just recall. The student can generalize to the main idea, infer, conclude, predict, and evaluate from imaged gestalts.

2. *Oral Language Comprehension*
   Visualizing/Verbalizing enables the student to receive, organize and comprehend oral language concepts. The student will respond to oral directions, humor, cause and effect relationships, and improve attention to oral language.

3. *Oral Language Expression*
   Visualizing/Verbalizing enables the student to receive, organize and express language concepts. The student is more able, organized, succinct, and fluent in verbalization. Imaged gestalts are the foundation from which he or she verbalizes.

4. *Written Language Expression*
   Visualizing/Verbalizing aids the student in writing skills. The student is more able to organize and structure the content of paragraphs and reports, due to improvement in oral language expression and awareness that writing creates images for the reader.

5. *Critical Thinking*
   The techniques embodied in the Visualizing/Verbalizing process aid in the development of critical thinking. *The approach is based on inquiry.* Once the student has developed an imaged gestalt for a concept, interpretive questions are asked regarding *main idea, inference, conclusion, prediction, and evaluation.* The process can be extended to cause-and-effect relationships in life situations.

The *Visualizing/Verbalizing* process is fairly simple and very successful if developed in the recommended series of specific steps. The imaging process moves from small units of language to larger units of language—first for a word, then to sentences, paragraphs, pages, and chapters.

I will present the *Visualizing/Verbalizing* process—referred to as *V/V*—in a personal writing style so that you will be able to practice visualizing as you read.

There will be sample dialogue and characters for you to experience through imagery. It is my hope that you will visualize and become a part of the sessions.

The following pages will present the treatment process for V/V in a one-to-one setting; however, Chapter 17 discusses classroom management and each summary page describes how to use the process with groups. As you read the dialogue, visualize the characters. The teacher is me...39-ish, female, vivacious, lots of dark hair, large dark eyes, obvious intelligence, warmth...and humility. The students are both male and female, of varying ages, with varying degrees of disability.

Chapter 3

Climate

The Reading Mother

You may have tangible wealth untold:
Caskets of jewels and coffers of gold.
Richer than I you can never be —
I had a Mother who read to me.

W ords change to "pictures" in your mind and those pictures change back to words to help you verbalize. This is what you are going to teach. The student must know what he or she will learn and why it is relevant. This is *setting the climate*. Your explanation should be brief but complete. Remember, your student has difficulty, whether severe or moderate, in comprehending language and it is easy to overexplain, become too wordy, or simply forget to notice the responses of individuals. Thus, assume your student has a severe language disorder and proceed to keep your explanation succinct. It is helpful to gesture in order to enhance imagery for the receiver of language.

The climate step must not be omitted. It is important that individuals know what they are doing and why they are doing it. They need to know how a task will be relevant to their life. Individuals of all ages will participate if they know how a task will help them and they have a *reason* to participate.

The following is an actual lesson from a climate session. The student is a girl named Linda, who is a member of the swim team with greenish-blond hair, average intelligence, and below-average grades. She is usually quiet.

---

sample lesson 1: Climate

Nanci: **"I'm going to explain** *what* **we are going to do and** *why* **we are going to do it. If we look at our brain from the top, we are looking down on the top of our**

head, and our brain looks something like this. (Draw a diagram of the brain.)

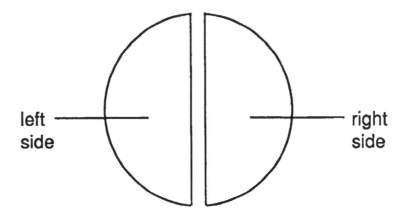

"We have two parts to our brain. A right side...here...and a left side...here. These are referred to as the right hemisphere and left hemisphere. (Touch the appropriate side of the diagram and even the student's head).

"These two parts of your brain do different things. When you visualize, or imagine, we think the right side of your brain works. It gets active like this. (Show brain activity by gesturing on your head and the student's head. Then make little dots on the right hemisphere of the diagram.)

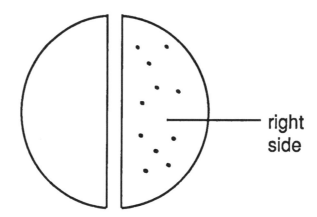

"When you talk, we think the left side of your brain works. It gets active, like this. (Again show the activity in the brain by gesturing on your head and making little dots on the left hemisphere of the diagram.)

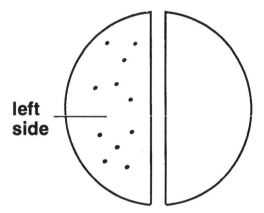

"I'm going to teach you how to use both sides of your brain. You will picture—imagine, visualize—and then you will talk about—verbalize — those pictures in your brain. (Show by arrows from one hemisphere to the other. Use the terms visualize and verbalize, in place of picture and talk about, as appropriate).

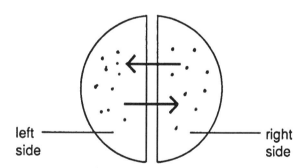

"As these two sides learn to work together, you will be able to understand and remember language better. For example,... Right now when you read, the words might go in one ear and out the other, like this:

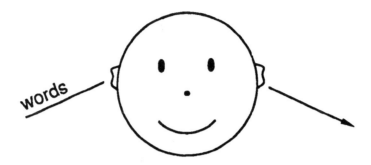

"But, if you make a picture of the words in your brain, an image, then the words will stay in your head in the form of pictures. This work will therefore help you remember what you read or hear."

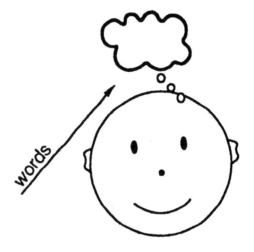

Verbalizing Explanation

If appropriate, extend the climate to an explanation of the need for verbalizing. Often this is helpful to older individuals with less severe dysfunction. If the individuals seem unable to follow or uninterested, save this discussion until later steps of V/V.

Your explanation stems from the premise that the purpose of the verbalizing aspect of V/V is twofold. First, the students' verbalizing is the means by which you know if the students are visualizing. It is your window to their brains. If they can describe an image, then you can be relatively confident imaging is occurring.

Second, the verbalizing activity results in more *concise* expressive language. The student is more able to organize thoughts and then verbalize those thoughts from images. Verbalizing is a critical aspect of cognition.

Continue extending the climate to discuss verbalizing.

Nanci: **"It is important for you to verbalize—talk about—your images because that is the only way I know if you are visualizing. For example:** (Draw two happy faces and label one the student and one yourself.)

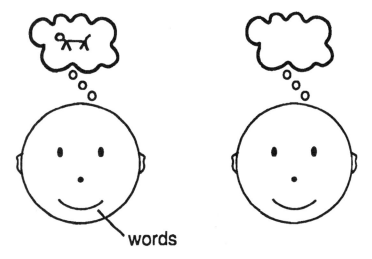

"You have a picture in your head about something like a cat. You can get that picture over to my head by using words to describe your picture. Then I'll have the same picture as you. (Complete the drawing:)

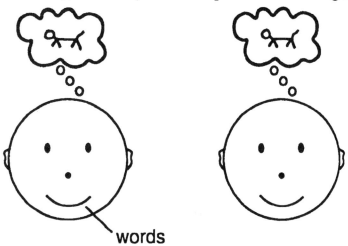

If working with an older individual, I might continue further: **"Also, as you talk about your images, you will become more comfortable with talking and expressing yourself. You will learn how to organize your words and talk to and with other people. When you can do this orally, aloud, then you will be able to write your thoughts too. That makes writing assignments easier, test taking easier, etc."**

Gesturing Explanation

It sometimes is helpful for individuals to shut their eyes when visualizing. This appears to enhance the activity in the right hemisphere. It is also important to enhance the activity in the left hemisphere by gesturing or pantomiming the verbalization. The following dialogue explains these concepts to the individual but adds length to the climate presentation and is therefore optional...perhaps to be used on another day.

Nanci: **"The right side of your brain has to image in order for you to improve your comprehension. So, it is very important that you create good, strong images in your brain. It may help if you close your eyes. This will stop the pictures you see with your eyes from interfering with the pictures you are seeing in your mind.**

"Just as you closed your eyes to help you visualize or imagine, you also may need to help yourself verbalize—talk. Watch me as I tell you a little story. What else is moving besides my mouth?

Gesturing... **"The propeller of the yellow airplane starts up, the airplane taxies down the runway, and then gets up speed and takes off into the air. It flies around for awhile, realizes it is running out of gas, turns around and comes back down for a bumpy landing.**

"Did you see me help myself talk? What was I using? Right, my hands and arms were moving to help me. That is gesturing."

Sometimes, I add contrast to this lesson by telling the same story without gesturing so that the individual can really **see** how the gesturing helped my verbalizing and his or her imaging. Obviously, you are free to omit, alter, or add to any of the above to suit your needs and experiences. Try to stay simple but descriptive. The dialogue above seems more lengthy in print than it does orally.

Reduced Climate Presentation

If working with young or severely disabled students, omit the above presentations and just draw a face and explain (while briefly diagramming) that:

1. They will learn to picture—imagine—things in their head.
2. Then they will talk about those images or pictures.
3. This will help them remember what they read and hear.

Summary of Climate

step 1

● *Keep the climate presentation short and succinct.*

Explain *what* will do:

1. Diagram right/left hemisphere of the brain.

2. Introduce concept of right hemisphere linked to imaging.

3. Introduce concept of left hemisphere linked to talking.

4. Show how both sides work together. Introduce the phrase "Visualizing and Verbalizing" or "picturing and talking about."

Explain *why* will do it:

5. Explain that visualizing improves the ability to understand/remember what we read/hear.

6. Explain that verbalizing improves the ability to express ourselves orally or in writing.

Optional:

7. Present a reduced climate presentation for young or severely disabled students.

8. Explain that gesturing is important because it enhances oral expression.

Chapter 4

Picture to Picture

This step needs to begin immediately following the climate. Don't wait. If time is an issue, use the reduced climate presentation so you can move the individual directly to this experience. At *picture to picture*, the individual looks at a given picture and describes that picture orally...thus creating a picture in the mind of the teacher.

This step is designed to give students practice verbalizing from a given picture prior to verbalizing from their images. Unfortunately, I was not aware of the importance of it in the early stages of developing the V/V process. When individuals had difficulty verbalizing, I assumed they couldn't visualize. Within a short time, however, I realized that I couldn't discern what was actually interfering. Was it that they couldn't visualize? Or was it that they couldn't verbalize?

The picture to picture level removes that question. Individuals are given practice verbalizing from a given picture. If they can verbalize from an actual picture but can't verbalize from their images, then you know that they aren't visualizing.

To begin, the student describes a simple picture that you cannot see and, ostensibly, have not seen. She is presented with the concept that her words will make "pictures" in your brain. You *question* to stimulate and refine her verbalization and introduce *structure words* as a guide for basic elements to be included in the description. Once the verbalization is completed—and you still haven't seen the given picture—you summarize and introduce the phrase: *"Your words make me picture..."* As you describe your image, the student may modify it by altering or adding more information. Having completed your description, you look at the given picture and discuss how it matched your image.

Along with the basic development of verbalization, this level also teaches a structure or framework from which to visualize and verbalize. The *structure words* assist the student in describing concepts of color, size, shape, number—physical and emotional aspects of images/thoughts. They also give her an opportunity to *sequentially reverbalize*.

47

An Overview of the Picture to Picture Steps

1. The student describes a given picture.

2. The teacher questions with choice and contrast.

3. The structure words are checked through for details and reverbalization by the student.

4. The teacher summarizes own image prior to seeing the given picture. Introduce the phrase, *"Your words made me picture...."* (You are describing your visualization and feeding back the student's verbalization.)

5. The teacher sees the picture. (The student shows you the picture and you compare your mental picture with the given picture.) If there is a discrepancy, rather than chastising, accept responsibility by saying, *"You know what, I didn't picture the...."*

Structure Words

The structure words provide the individual with a guide or structure for including detail in the verbalization and visualization. They may be introduced one or two at a time—or all at once—depending on the needs of your student(s).

There are two categories of structure words: gross and fine.

> *gross:* **what**[1] **size**[2] **color**[3] **number**[4] **shape**[5] **where**[6]

> *fine:* **movement**[7] **mood**[8] **background**[9] **perspective**[10] **when**[11] **sound**[12]

The structure words are numbered for their relative importance to gestalt imagery. The numbering resulted from observation of teachers, reading specialists, speech therapists, special day teachers, etc. in numerous V/V classes. During the practice section of the class, teachers frequently had students attend to the *background* structure word prior to attending to the *what* structure word. This drew the student away from the gestalt and the sequential elements that would describe the gestalt. For example, the student should describe the *what*—usually the largest item in the picture—and then describe details concerning the *what* such as its *size, color, shape,* etc. It is important to have the student give fairly detailed descriptions of the *what* and then move to *background* and *perspective,* etc. Often an individual with a weakness in imaging gestalts will describe the parts first, rather than the gestalt. Attending to a sequential use of the structure words can help correct this.

The structure words in the appendix can be cut out and printed on card stock. Or you can just write them on 3 x 5 cards. All are self-explanatory in the "gross" category, but the "fine" group may need some explanation. For example, *Mood* refers to the emotional element of the picture, such as happiness, sadness, anger, etc. *Movement* refers to any activity in the picture. *Background* refers to any background in the picture! *Perspective* refers to how the student is viewing the picture, ("Are we looking at this image from above, up really close, or far away?"). Perspective seems to be particularly important when individuals are creating their own images. I often image whole scenes from an aerial position and then zoom in closer for detailed images. However, students frequently seem to have difficulty visualizing whole scenes from above. Instead, they tend to be too close and can only image parts.

When refers to either era or gross time, such as morning, night, day, etc. *Sound* refers to any sounds the individual can hear from the images depicted. Although sound may not develop until later, some individuals spontaneously add the aspect of sound to their images perhaps indicating an intense image experience.

The following lesson continues with Linda, the swimmer with the synthetic looking hair.

sample lesson 2: Introducing Structure Words

Nanci: **"Let's begin visualizing and verbalizing. I want you to use words to describe this picture. Your words will make me have a picture in my brain. You verbalize/talk and I'll visualize/picture."** (While you say this, gesture to the diagram you used in the climate presentation. Or gesture from her mouth to your head).

Give the student a simple, *colored* picture. Have her describe some of it. The verbalization may be limited and lacking refinement. Introduce the structure words as below to provide essential elements of detail.

Nanci: **"There were certain things you talked about that helped me get a strong picture in my mind. First it is important to tell me *what* the picture is about —not a dog, or an elephant, but a girl.**

Place the *what* structure word on the table before her.

"If you describe the girl in this picture only as a "girl," will I know if she has green short hair or three legs? The picture in my mind has to match your picture.

"If you say, 'a little girl' that changes my picture... We will call that *size*. Your word, 'little', made me picture the size of the girl in the picture. It was important; otherwise, I might picture a real big girl."

Place the *size* structure word in front of her. You may return to or make a new diagram of the two faces from the climate presentation...illustrate a little girl in the student's head and a big girl in your head, stick figures suffice.

Proceed to put down other structure words, describing the importance of each one. For example, "*Color* helps me picture the color of her skin, the color of her hair, her dress, her shoes, the sky, etc."

Decide how many of the structure words you want to introduce and explore the concept of each. I usually introduce all of them at once, but if your students are very young or very language disabled, choose to introduce only the first three: *what, size, color*. Add more each session. How much or how little depends upon your diagnosis.

If your student(s) cannot decode yet, read the words and illustrate their concept on the *back* of the card. For example, the structure word *what* may have the printed word **what** on one side and question marks on the other. *Size* may have stick figures of different sizes. *Color* may have different colors.

Choosing a Picture

The picture to picture level is necessary for all ages and your choice of the given picture is critical. **It is extremely important to use pictures with few details.** Use this simple criteria when choosing pictures:

- One central figure
- Very little detail
- None or very little background.
- Color

The simplicity of the picture is the key. If the picture is too detailed the lesson becomes lengthy, complicated, and unproductive. Sample pictures are provided in the appendix. Be sure to color them! Don't have students describe black and white pictures when doing the V/V program. While in Australia teaching V/V classes, I went to a very good speech/language center that was using V/V with all students. However, "figure-ground" problems had been created by students describing black and white pictures. The sample pictures in the appendix are meant to be copied and *colored*, and are only samples. Additional simple pictures can be found in vocabulary kits, coloring books, magazine advertisements, etc. "Age-appropriateness" does not seem to matter. I have college students describe simple primary pictures. The goal is to develop refined detailed verbalization. If students know that, then any simple, colored picture will do and will be relevant to the task.

Questioning

Questioning can directly stimulate imagery and thus establish a sensory-cognitive base for comprehension and analytical thinking.

When I became aware that some individuals didn't image gestalts easily, I thought I could just *tell* them to visualize. "I'll read you a story and you picture it in your mind." Soon I realized that stimulating imagery through prodding or telling just wasn't effective. It didn't work. Faces looked back at me...blank faces...faces trying to please...apologetic faces...curious faces...faces that just couldn't do what I *told* them to do.

So, if I couldn't command them to image, perhaps I could *question* them to image. Questions. Questions to give choices for images. Questions to stimulate contrasting images. Questions to interact and direct imagery. It worked. I could stimulate imagery with questions!

The basic questioning technique means asking a question that requires more than a yes/no response and offers choice and contrast (See chapter 15 for details on How to Question). Note my specific questioning technique with Linda in the next *Picture to Picture* lesson. The goal is to develop *her verbalizing* so I use a question to stimulate it directly by saying, *"What should I see for the...?"* This specific language reinforces that she must refine her verbalizing to create images in my mind. In the next step of V/V—*Word Imaging*—the goal is to develop her visualizing. Then my question will be, *"What do you see for the...?"*

---

sample lesson 3: Picture to Picture

Nanci: **"You're going to describe another picture that I won't see. Your words will create a picture in my mind...I'll visualize what you say. When you are** through, without looking at the picture, I'll tell you what I visualized. Then we will check and see how good you were at describing the picture."

Linda: "Should I use those structure words?"

Nanci: "First just describe the picture as best you can, then we'll go back and check through the structure words to decide if you've included all of them."

Linda begins to describe a given—simple, colored—picture of a young black girl playing a toy piano.

Linda: "There is a girl...and...she is playing a piano."

Nanci: "That's a good start. Help me picture the girl better. Is she big, little...?"

Linda: "She's little."

Nanci: "Little like this...(gesturing to real small size between fingers)...or young?"

Linda: "Young."

Nanci: "OK. Help me know how young to picture her. Is she young like a baby, young like a two year old, young like a...?"

Linda: "Young like about 5 years old."

Nanci: "Oh. Now my picture is getting better. I see a young girl. Is she a white girl, black girl, brown...."

Linda: (Interrupting). "She's black."

Nanci: "OK. That helps me. I see a young black girl, about 5 years old, playing a piano. Does she have clothes on...or not?"

Linda: "Yeah. She's got on a dress...a red dress."

Nanci: "Short dress? Long dress? Short sleeves? What should I see for her dress? Give me as much information as you can."

Linda: "It's a short dress...the sleeves are sort of...puffy...and it has dots on it...white dots."

Nanci: "Good, now my picture is getting even better. Should I see big white dots or...."

Linda: (interrupting) "No. Little white dots and there is a bow in back. Also, she has on shoes...black shoes...and white socks."

Nanci: "Really good. Now, does she have any hair?"

Linda: (Laughs...finally) "Yeah. She has black curly hair...it's sort of short but not too short."

Nanci: "Good. My picture is getting better and better. Now, what position should I see her in? Is she standing on one leg or perhaps standing on her hands and playing the piano with her toes...how shall I picture her?"

Linda: (Little laugh) "She is sitting on the floor...sort of sitting on her knees and playing the piano with her hands. There's a book open on the piano, too."

Nanci: "Boy, I have a strange picture. How can she sit on her knees and reach the piano with her hands? Is it...?"

Linda: (Interrupting) "It's a little piano...like a toy piano and it's right in front of her."

She continues describing the color, size, shape, etc. of the piano. I mentally file through the structure words to help me know which questions to ask. For example, next I ask about *where*, then *movement* and *mood*. As our interaction begins to wane, we check through the structure words so she can get more experience verbalizing and can add details to her description.

Nanci: "Good job. Now let's use those structure words. I'll put them out in front of you and you can start with number 1—*what*— and just quickly tell me a little bit about each one. For example, did you tell me the *what*?"

Linda: "Yeah. I told you it is a little girl playing a toy piano."

Nanci: "Good. Turn that card over and go to the next one—*size*. Did you tell me anything about *size*?"

Linda: "Yeah. I told you the girl is about 5 years old, she's got sort of short hair...hmmm, the piano is small."

Nanci: "Right. Turn that card over. How about *color*?"

We continue checking through all the structure words. Realizing we didn't include a few in the description, we simply add their specific details now. We finish with a complete description and proceed to complete the lesson.

Nanci: "Good job. Your words have given me a really good picture. Let's see how I did. I'll describe my picture to you and you check me. Here we go. *Your words made me picture* a young black girl, about 5 years old, playing a toy piano. She has short black curly hair. I can see the side of her face and she has a little nose, one brown eye showing, a rosy cheek, and her mouth is open like she is singing. Also, she has on a red dress with white—little white—dots. The dress is short with short puffed-out sleeves. She has on black shoes and white socks. Are the socks long, like up to her knees, or short?"

Linda: "Short...and sort of scrunched down."

Nanci: "OK. I had them up to her knees. I'll just change my picture. Now, let's see. She is sitting on her knees and...."

I continue to give my image back to her in as much detail as I can recall. This is not as difficult as you might think since, although I haven't looked at the picture yet with Linda, I have seen it before! After all, I chose these pictures initially and knew immediately which picture she was describing. It helped my imaging, but more important, it helped my questioning.

Nanci: "How did I do? Did I get everything?"

Linda: "Almost. You forgot to tell me that she has a bow on her dress."

Nanci: "Oh, that's right. Know what? I didn't put that in my picture so I forgot it! I'll just add it right now. Anything else?"

Linda: "No."

Nanci: "Good job—let me see the picture!"

We look at the picture together. She described most of it, but left out another book on top of the piano.

Nanci: "You did a good job. Know what? I didn't picture this book on top of the piano."

I owned the error by saying, "I didn't picture"...rather than "You didn't tell me about...." Consequently, the lesson ended positively rather negatively.

Summary

Continue the *picture to picture* lessons until the individual is confidently describing given pictures and is including the concepts of the structure words. Note that the structure words will aid the teacher in questioning as well as aid the individual in verbalizing.

The picture to picture level may require only a few minutes or a few lessons, again depending on your student. However, it is important to include it with individuals, even if only to evaluate their ability to verbalize and familiarize them with the structure words for later use.

As I stated at the beginning of this chapter, I originally did not include this step with every student. This anecdote will help you remember why *you should include picture to picture practice with every student.*

I was working with a fifth-grade boy. We had previously developed his word recognition and word attack by using the Lindamood Auditory Discrimination in Depth (ADD) program. He was now decoding above his grade level. His comprehension had appeared only modestly weak in the original diagnostic testing. However, he had gained a couple of years in decoding and was now reading paragraphs at a much higher level than was possible only months before. Whereas he previously had comprehended lower level material with ease, he was now reading higher level material and experiencing difficulty. We initiated Visualizing and Verbalizing.

Gary was verbal in most situations. Precisely because of his verbal ability, I thought his dysfunction was moderate and omitted the *picture to picture* level. I moved immediately into the next steps of *known nouns* and *sentence by sentence* and presented the structure words at that time. I was in a hurry.

Weeks passed and Gary was having much difficulty describing his images. Day after day, the tutor noted "much difficulty imaging...much difficulty verbalizing." After two or three weeks of frustration, I looked back in the clinical notes to my original introduction of the V/V process. It was then I realized that I had omitted the picture to picture level. So, for a week, I had him back up and describe given pictures to me, using the structure words to monitor and check his verbalization. Interestingly enough, he had difficulty just looking at a given picture and describing it. Naturally he had difficulty describing his images!

After only a week or so of picture to picture practice, he was able to extend to verbalizing his images. His visualization seemed improved since he could now verbalize more fluently. Within weeks, he was having very positive sessions and moved from third- and fourth-grade material into fifth-grade material. Within another month he was visualizing and verbalizing from sixth-grade material and we were beginning to apply this technique to his school work. The picture to picture step didn't cure Gary, but it was a significant part of the whole process.

Gesturing

We must unconsciously know that visualizing is important to language comprehension or why would we gesture as we talk? Gestures serve two purposes: they support the images of the sender, and they help build the images of the receiver. As I gesture, I am linking my images with my words. As my listener sees my gestures, he or she is linking my words with his or her images.

Some individuals seem to gesture automatically. Good storytellers use lots of gestures. In fact, they often use more than gestures to help us experience their story. They do sound effects, body movements, facial expressions, etc. "We drove the jeep over a bumpy, mountain road (hands on an imaginary steering wheel, body simulating bouncing while making slight auditory impression of a jeep motor), ...and then suddenly, there was a loud bang and the jeep swerved off to the right (steering wheel motion)...I slammed on the brakes (foot motion)"...etc.

Although many individuals naturally augment their verbalization with gestures, some individuals with language comprehension difficulty don't even move their hands or fingertips while talking. They talk and gesture very little. With few or vague images, there may be little sensory information from which they can gesture or verbalize. They often seem wrapped in a cloak of no movements, no expression, and no language.

Practicing gesturing is optional and simple. Try two steps: gesture a simple object and a simple movement.

Gesturing a single object:

1. Begin with something concrete in front of the student such as a shape-object: ball, triangle, square. For example, the student feels a medium sized ball then uses her hands to gesture it. Continue with other objects that can be easily felt and gestured.

2. Continue by gesturing objects from memory such as an ice-cream cone, a cup, a Christmas tree shape, an umbrella, and a hat.

Gesturing a movement:

1. Gesturing extends to movement with exaggeration. Pantomime a movement-word and extend to a movement-sentence.

Some movement words to gesture:
- *walking:* student shows walking with two fingers for legs
- *running:* student shows running as above, only faster
- *jumping:* student again uses fingers and hand, not own body!
- *flying:* student uses hand in closed-finger position

Some movement sentences to gesture:
- The boy ran up the hill (fingers running upward).
- The girl throws the ball.
- The elephant trunk was swinging back and forth.
- He drank a glass of water very slowly...then very quickly.

The above step is optional and primarily used with severe language handicapped students. Keep in mind that these students might have such limited imagery that gesturing the sentences will be difficult. You may then need to begin to develop gesturing and visualizing/verbalizing simultaneously. These areas all support one another. If you choose not to practice gesturing as a separate step, you can easily incorporate it into other lessons.

Practice Picture to Picture

Practice is obviously important and the amount of it depends on your student and your diagnosis. A criterion for how long to practice any given step is about 80% accuracy or...until the student is *fairly comfortable* with the task. In the initial steps of V/V, the *climate* and *picture to picture* reinforcement are initiated in the same lesson. Continue at the picture to picture level until the student is fairly apt at verbalizing from a given picture and introduce the next step of word imaging while picture to picture lessons are stabilizing. The steps overlap. In the same session that a student is practicing verbalizing from a given picture, she also may be practicing verbalizing from her own image.

Picture to Picture

1. Linda describes a picture.

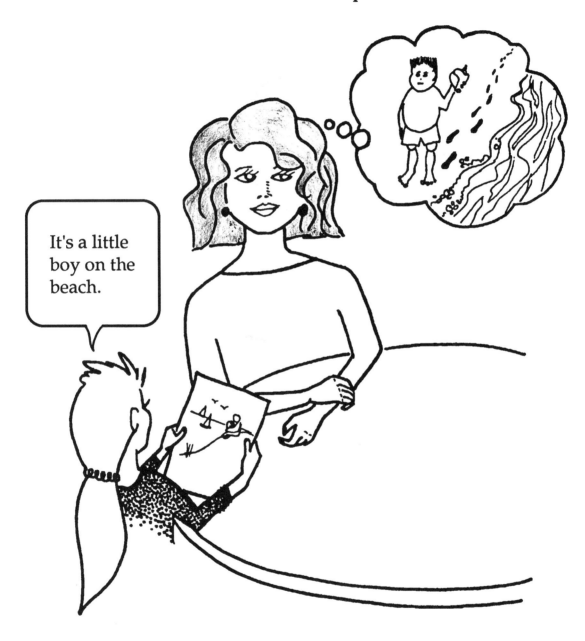

2. **Nanci questions.**

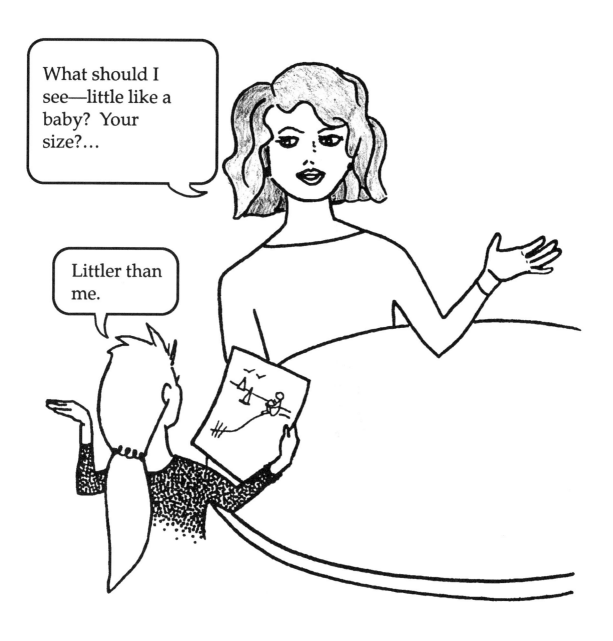

3. Linda checks through the structure words.

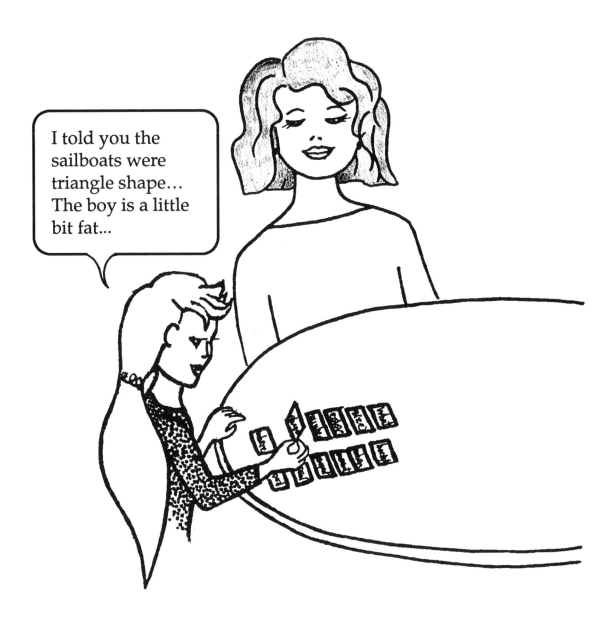

4. Nanci summarizes.

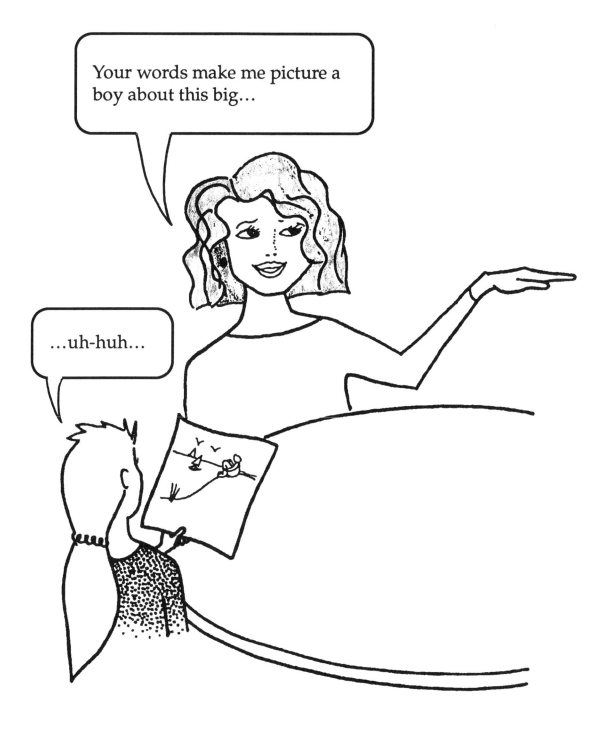

Summary of Picture to Picture

step 2

Objective: The student will be able to give a *detailed* verbal description of a simple picture. ***Present structure words:*** *what, size, color, number, shape, where, movement, mood, background, perspective, when, sound.*

1. The student verbally describes a simple, colored picture.

2. The teacher questions with choice and contrast to develop and refine verbalizing.

3. The student checks through the structure words, quickly reverbalizing each element.

4. The teacher summaries, using the phrase: *"Your words made me picture...."*

5. The teacher sees the picture and discusses it with the student.

6. Use simple, colored pictures with little detail and background.

7. Practice picture to picture until the student is comfortable with the task. Overlap to next step—*Word Imaging*—while continuing to practice.

8. Practice gesturing of simple objects and sentences—optional.

9. **Group Instruction:**
   Small groups of 3 to 5 are recommended. The group represents a collective individual so the interaction is similar to one-to-one. For example: Show a picture to all 5 students. Randomly choose students to describe the picture and check through structure words. This allows all students to participate and you only receive (visualize) one picture.

Chapter 5

Word Imaging

Now that the individual is able to verbalize from a given picture, V/V moves to **visualizing**. The goal is to develop gestalt imagery. The visualizing activity begins with the smallest "part" of language—a single word.

At the *word imaging* level, individuals describe their visualization of a single word. Similar in format to *picture to picture*, the focus is now on visualizing rather than verbalizing. The teacher questions, the structure words are used for details and reverbalization, the student monitors, adjusts, and refines her imaging and verbalizing. She creates an image in the mind of the teacher who then summarizes it to complete the stimulation.

As expected, there is a range in students' imaging ability. Although some individuals find it very difficult, it is believed that everyone *can* image. It's that the images may range from very strong and vivid to very weak and vague. For example, individuals with difficulty imaging report that the images are dim, don't have color or motion, and seem to float by very quickly. Conversely, individuals with good imaging ability report that the images are vivid and intense and may even include auditory and olfactory sensations. I have had clinical sessions with professional people—doctors, teachers, businessmen, as well as college students—who found it very difficult to visualize. Although we don't consider these people "learning disabled," many had language comprehension/expression problems to some degree and were impaired in their ability to create images.

Considering the above, expect that visualizing will be difficult, not automatic, for your student. He or she will need stimulation, interaction, practice, and patience.

Visualizing an Object

Word imaging usually begins with a word that is very familiar to the student; a pet or something in the student's own home or environment. However, even with a ginger first step such as this, some individuals can't understand what you mean by an image or visualization. They think you want them to see something very bold on their eyelids when they close their eyes or they think you mean an image that is exactly like a clear picture on a movie screen or TV monitor. You can expect some confusion as well as the need for clarification about what it means to visualize. Because of this, I have included the following sample lesson that I use only when the student has severe difficulty understanding what it means to image. This lesson begins by having the student actually look at an object and close her eyes to be able to still "see" that same object.

sample lesson 4: Visualization of an Object

Nanci: **"Now, you are going to practice visualizing. Look at that chair. Close your eyes and imagine what it looks like. Can you still see it in your imagination? If not, look at it again, go over and feel the chair as if you were a blind person. See if you can imagine it."**

If you need to, practice this activity with other objects in the room or bring in objects. Have the student tell you about the object with her eyes closed. Try to get the student to use the gross structure words to help you visualize what she is picturing. Remember, don't do this activity unless you feel the student can't image something personal.

Personal Imaging

If you needed to include object imaging, you should proceed to *personal images* within minutes. *Personal imaging* allows the student to recall something familiar such as a pet. Initially try to pick something that is personal but also simple to describe. Although family members may be personal, they are not always easy to describe. The same is true for an individual's living space, such as a bedroom or home. Choose a part of the living space to visualize and verbalize and keep the verbalization simple by not asking questions that will lead to a very lengthy description.

The lesson below continues with the swimmer, Linda.

sample lesson 5: Personal Images

Nanci: **"Let's give your brain practice imaging. You need to talk to me about the picture in your brain so I can see it, too. This is like what you did when you had a picture in front of you, only now the picture is in your brain.**

"Do you have a pet? Imagine—visualize—that pet. Can you see it? Close your eyes if you need to.

"Now, help me to see it by describing it with words. First describe your image as best you can—then we'll use the structure words to see if you included all the details."

The structure words should *not* be in front of the student.

Note: Occasionally a student may verbalize at this level fairly well, but generally it is necessary to question with choice and contrast. Remember the object of this is to stimulate visualizing so your questions should be phrased, *"What do you see for the...*not "What should I see...."

Linda: **"My pet is a dog."**

Nanci: **"I imagine a little, purple dog...is that right?"**

Linda: (laughs)... **"No, he is a big white dog."**

Nanci: **"OK, now your words make me picture a big white dog."**

Note: The student may be willing to stop right here. However, notice the refinement of visualization and language as we develop *detailed imagery*.

Nanci: **"What kind of big white dog should I visualize? Do you know what type of dog you have? A dog with real smooth hair or lots of hair like a poodle or sheepdog?"**

Linda: **"Lots of hair...he is a husky."**

Nanci: **"Now your words are really helping me get a good image. Let's keep going. What do you see for his tail? Does he have a tail like a little rabbit...a little fluffy tail?"**

Linda: **"No, he has a curly tail."**

Nanci: **"A curly tail...like a cork- screw... like this (gesturing) is that what you see?"**

Linda: (laughs)..."No, like a half circle, going up. When he is in a good mood it just pops right up. When he is not... it just goes down."

The student is beginning to do a little gesturing. I continue to develop *detailed images* as I stimulate further.

Nanci: **"I'm picturing a big white husky-type dog with a curly tail but...no face! His face is just all white in my imagination. What do you see?"**

Linda: (Interrupts)... **"No, he has a nose...a black nose and eyes."**

Nanci: **"Big blue eyes?"**

Linda: **"No, big, brown eyes."**

Nanci: **"Do you see real big eyes like this (gesture)?"**

Linda: **"No, they are about this big (gesturing)."**

Nanci: **"Ok, I see his eyes...and nose...and great big donkey ears!"**

Linda: **"No! No, he has little ears like this (gesturing)."**

Note: The dialogue was taken from an actual session in which I had to question to help her create an image. My technique of describing something unexpected, a contrast, such as "donkey ears," kept the student attending, involved, and hopefully added levity to the session.

Linda was very unexpressive, due either to weak imaging or weak verbalizing or both. She seemed satisfied with skeletal descriptions so I continued questioning.

Nanci: **"Does he have a collar? I have him pictured with a collar, but I can't be sure that it is the same kind of collar that you see."**

Linda: **"It's a...just a regular collar...a nice blue one."**

Nanci: **"Oh, blue! I had a brown collar visualized!"**

Linda: **"No, this way it stands out more."**

We interact further. I question to stimulate the intensity and details of her imaging. When I feel we have developed a fairly good personal image, I move to checking through the structure words. This develops both her visualizing and her verbalizing.

Nanci: **"Good job. Now let's check through the structure words to see if we have all the details."**

Place the structure words face up, sequentially, on the table.

"This structure word says *what*. Did you tell me *what* you were picturing?"

Linda: **"I was picturing my dog...a husky."**

Nanci: **"Good. Turn the *what* card over and keep going through the rest of them."**

Linda: **"*Size*. Yeah. I told you he was a big white dog with a long tail.** She turns over the *size* card.

"*Color*. Yeah. I told you he is a white dog and he has brown eyes—big brown eyes." She turns over the *color* card and continues through the others until she gets to *movement*.

"I didn't tell you about any *movement*. He is just standing. Should I make him move?"

Nanci: **"If you want. Can you have him do something like scratch fleas, jump up...?"**

Linda: (Interrupts) **"Biting at flies! He is biting at flies in the air. He does that a lot."**

Nanci: **"Good. What are you picturing for that?"**

Linda proceeds to describe her dog biting at flies—mouth snapping open, quick head movements—and adds more information when she gets to the *mood* structure word. She—*we*—have created a vivid, detailed image. (I visualize lots of little synapses occurring in her brain).

Nanci: **"OK. Now, let me tell you my image. Your words make me picture a big, white husky dog with a curly tail...Up when he is happy...down when he is not. I can see it moving. He has a bright blue collar, black nose, brown eyes, and..."** I proceed to give her a detailed verbalization of my image, she corrects, adds, or changes information.

Known Noun Imaging

The *known noun* level is very important because it is here that we establish detailed imagery for a single word. The word is something known but not necessarily

69

personally experienced by the student, so choose words that are in her realm of knowledge. Words such as Indian, clown, and boat are familiar, high imagery nouns.

Here are a few good choices:

clown	Santa Claus
Christmas tree	monkey
Indian	fire truck
doll	butterfly
Mickey Mouse	airplane
cowboy	owl
banana split	snake
dog	horse
cat	tiger
elephant	flower

Poor choices would be words without differentiating characteristics. Generic words such as "chair," "sofa," "sky," tree" don't lend themselves to detailed imagery.

The following lesson continues with Linda.

sample lesson 6: Known Noun Imaging

Begin the lesson by giving her a word to visualize. She images the word concept and describes the image using the structure words to focus language and provide details.

Nanci: **"I am going to say a word to you and I want you to visualize the word...not the letters of the word, but the thought of the word. Then you will describe your image so that I will have the same picture in my head.**

"Here is your word...*boat.*"

Linda: **"I see it."**

Nanci: **"Good. Now use words to help me picture what you are seeing in your mind."**

Linda: **"A boat... I see a boat."**

Nanci: **"A little tiny boat for the bathtub?"**

Linda: **"No, a big boat."**

Nanci: **"Good. You're telling me the size to picture. When you say big, should I see real, real big...like a huge ocean ship...or...?"**

Linda: **"No, a boat like on a lake."**

Note: You may want to ask the student to close her eyes and relax to strengthen her image. However, sometimes individuals are reluctant to do so, perhaps feeling threatened. If so, just encourage them to block out visual stimulation from their surroundings by putting their hands over their eyes or resting their head on their hands, covering their eyes.

Nanci: **"Good. I now know that this boat is not as big as a huge ship and not as small as a toy boat. But give me more information about the size... What do you see? Is it like a row boat...a sail boat...a motor boat...?"**

Note: Remember to give the student choices when you question. This very often will create or focus an image. Again this dialogue is from a session I had with Linda...and I was not sure that she actually visualized a specific boat until I gave her the choices. But, does it matter? *She is visualizing now.*

Linda: **"It's a sailboat."**

Nanci: **"Good. Now your picture is getting better. What color do you see for the boat...red, yellow, blue, pink...?"**

Note: Remember in the initial stages of V/V ask specific questions rather than general questions. They direct conscious attention to create, clarify, or refine an image.

Linda: **"It is yellow."**

Nanci: **"What part of the boat is yellow? Do you see the sails or the body yellow?"** (Note that I didn't *assume* imaging.)

Linda: **"The body part...the sail is white."**

Nanci: "You're doing a good job of visualizing Your words make me picture a yellow sailboat with white sails. What color do you see for the water and the sky? Do you see any people in the boat? Tell me more."

Linda: "The lake is greenish and the sky is blue."

Nanci: "A sunny day? Are there any clouds in the sky?"

Linda: "I don't know."

The ever feared "I don't know" response! This could have occurred at anytime in this session and it is probable that it will occur again. Here is one way to get beyond it.

Nanci: "Close your eyes and try to see the kind of day in your mind. Can you?"

Linda: "I guess so... "

Nanci: "This is your picture...you can make it any kind of day you want. You can make it sunny and bright with some white, puffy clouds in the sky or you can make it dark and rainy with a gray sky."

Linda: "Sunny with blue sky and some white clouds."

Nanci: "OK. I have that, too. Can you describe what you see?"

Note: If you have helped the student create an image, then check to be sure that she really "sees" it and isn't just restating or paraphrasing your words.

This interaction continued until we had generated a fairly strong image. As I decided how much to include, I kept in mind the energy of the lesson. The structure words are next so she can get more detailed imagery and practice verbalizing.

Nanci: "Good job! Now let's check through the structure words.

Place structure words in front of her.

"Did you tell me *what* you were seeing?"

Linda: "Yeah, I'm picturing a yellow and white sailboat."

Nanci: "Good. Turn that card over. Did you tell me *size*?"

Linda: "Yeah. I told you the size of the boat...it is a regular sail boat."

Nanci: "Not a toy sail boat, right? What about the size of the people in the boat?"

Linda: "Yeah. I told you there were two girls about my size."

Nanci: "Good. Turn that card over and keep going."

Linda: "*Color*—There is lots of color...yellow boat...white sails...blue sky...red bathing suits...greenish blue water. (She turns over the cards as she goes.)

Number—Hmmm. Two people on the boat, some clouds...one boat.

Where—On a lake.

Background—Just a big lake, nothing around it, just blue sky.

Movement—The sailboat is moving around because it is windy."

Nanci: "Moving around real fast (gesturing) or sort of slow?"

Linda: "Slow...like this... sort of...(gesturing)."

Mood—Hmmm...the girls are happy!

Perspective—I don't know."

Nanci: "How are you looking at your picture? From above and looking down... from far away...from sort of up close...?"

Linda: "Sort of far away."

When—I don't know."

Nanci: "Is it in early morning or late in the day, almost night...or?"

Linda: "It's morning. It's not getting dark or anything yet."

Nanci: (I concluded the session by summarizing the image she had created in my mind.) "Your words made me picture a sailboat on the ocean. It is sunny and bright outside with some white puffy clouds in the sky. The sailboat is yellow with white sails and two people are on board in red bathing suits... the lake is greenish blue..." We finished on a very positive note. We

73

shared, we experienced, and we began to stimulate a sensory cognitive base for reasoning and comprehension.

Fantasy Imaging

Fantasy imaging is helpful for intensifying images and easily included with known noun imaging as another means of developing *detailed imagery*. Remember it is critical in the early stages of the V/V process to develop *detailed imagery* to intensify the brain activity for visualizing. Without questioning for details such as color, size, shape, and background, the individual may continue to have weak, fleeting images and consequently little progress in the entire V/V process.

Observe individuals' reactions to fanciful images. Laughter or reaction to a ridiculous image indicates visualizing and vice versa.

---

sample lesson 7: Fantasy Imaging

Linda has had a number of sessions at the *known noun* level by this time.

Nanci: "Now, let's visualize the word elephant. You might want to check through the structure words in your mind to think with."

Linda: "OK. I see an elephant, a gray elephant...a big, gray elephant."

Nanci: "Good. Your words made me picture the size and color of the elephant. Right now my elephant is standing on one foot...squirting water at me."

Linda: "No, my elephant is standing on all four legs!"

Nanci: "Are we looking at the elephant from his front...like is he here (gesturing an elephant directly in front of me) and are we looking at his ears, eyes, and trunk...or are we behind the elephant...or to the side?"

Linda: "I am seeing the side of the elephant."

Nanci: "Good. It would help me visualize if you would remember to use gestures to show me that. Where do you see his head, ears, tail? Describe them as you go."

Linda proceeds to describe in response to my questions. I ask for more detail now:

Nanci: **"What do you see for the elephant's face. Does he have on dark glasses? Let's get some more detail."**

Linda: (Laughs) **"No glasses but he has eyes and a trunk."**

Nanci: **"Little, tiny, blue eyes?"**

Linda: **"OK! No, big brownish eyes and a big ear here...and a trunk."**

Urge her to gesture. I often take students' hands and help them see and feel the size of an ear or the shape of an elephant's trunk. We checked through the structure words, I gave her a summary, and then included fantasy imaging.

Nanci: **"Good. Your words gave me that good picture that I just described to you. Let's have some fun with our elephant. Close your eyes. Make him pink with a little red hat on his head...See him sitting in the sun at a swimming pool...diving off a diving board...with a big splash. Can you see it?"**

Linda described what she imaged, gesturing and smiling. We included sunglasses... holding a yellow umbrella in his trunk...on roller skates.

Summary

The word imaging level develops detailed imagery for the smallest unit of language —a word. Individuals with a severe language handicap may have difficulty with concepts such as down, up, between, under, front, back, and those basic language concepts can be taught at this level. The goal is to make words as real as possible by using imagery to experience the concept of a word. With imagery, words can be experienced vicariously. Detailed, intensified imagery enables individuals to experience concepts with sensory input that in turn enables them to store and retrieve information for use in oral and written comprehension and expression.

As the process proceeds, the student requires less and less specific questioning. Later, she may not need to check through the structure words since the characteristics they represent will be in her mind and she will automatically include their elements. She will be generating to the attributes of size, color, number, background, when, movement, mood, etc., without direct stimulation. You will question less and it will be important to ask opened-ended questions. In fact, if you continue to ask directed questions, she may rely on your thinking and images rather than spontaneously creating her own. Your goal is to be able to say, "Good, tell me more about what you see..." When this happens, you are ready to move to the next step of *sentence by sentence imaging.*

Practice Word Imaging

Practice with *known nouns* continues until the individual becomes fairly confident and fluent at visualizing and verbalizing images. *Watch for the student's eyes to look up, or defocus, as an indication of visualization.*

It is important to practice word imaging. Practice until there is approximately 80% accuracy and fair confidence with a task. It is also important to maintain interest and energy in the sessions. An overlap of steps assists in that. Remember, word imaging can be introduced while picture to picture lessons are stabilizing. Thus, in the same lesson the student may be practicing verbalizing from a given picture as well as practicing verbalizing from her own image. The time to complete the steps depends on the student, but an average student would be comfortable with these two steps within a few days or a few weeks.

Word Imaging

1. Linda is presented with a "known noun" to visualize and verbalize.

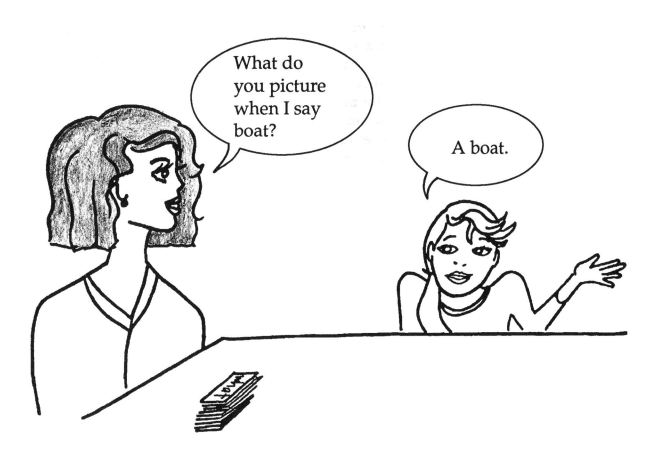

2. Nanci questions to develop detailed imagery.

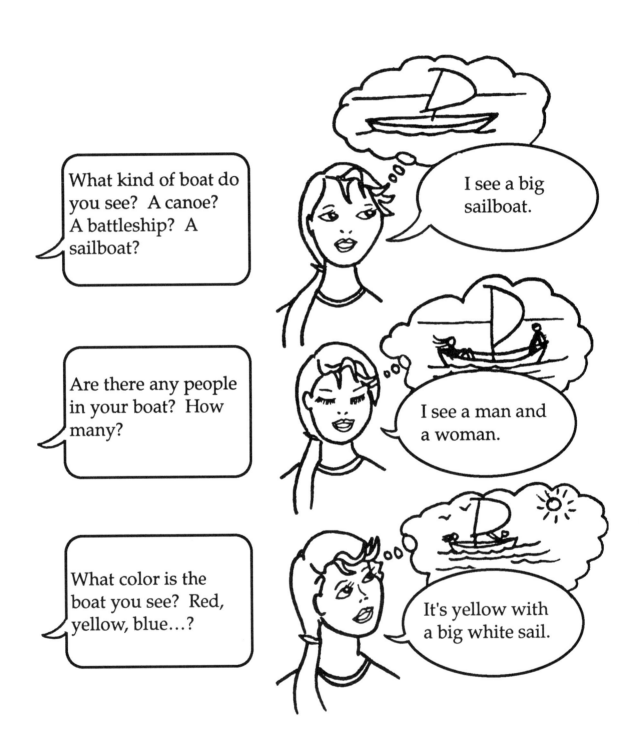

3. Nanci summarizes.

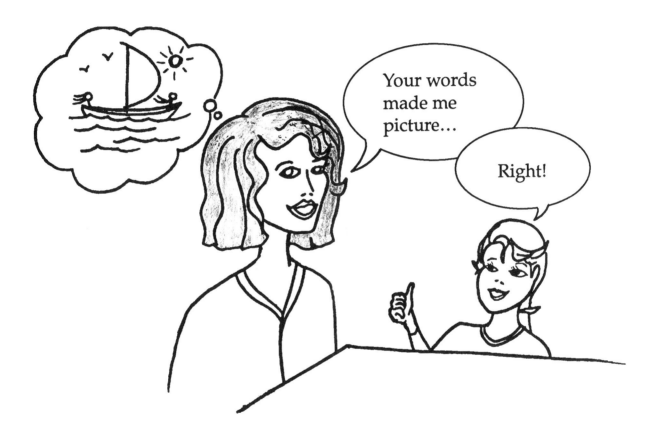

Summary of Word Imaging

step 3

Objective: The student will be able to visualize and verbalize, with *detail*, a single word.

1. **Object Imaging** (optional)

    a. Object imaging is for students who have difficulty understanding what it is to image.
    b. The student looks at an object, closes eyes, recalls and describes image.

2. **Personal Imaging** (not optional but only do one or two)

    a. The student recalls, images, and describes something personal but simple such as a pet, room, toy, etc.
    b. The teacher questions with choice and contrast.
    c. The structure words are checked through for details and reverbalization.
    d. The teacher gives a verbal summary using the phrase: "Your words made me picture...."

3. **Known Noun Imaging** (*not optional*)

    a. The student visualizes and verbalizes a noun. The word should be familiar as well as high in imagery.
    b. The teacher questions specifically with choice and contrast to develop detailed imagery.
    c. The structure words are checked through for details and reverbalization.
    d. If student has been given a choice, have the student describe the image to be sure not restating or paraphrasing.
    e. Request gesturing.
    f. Conclude session with a verbal summary using the phrase: *"Your words made me picture...."*
    g. Practice this step until very confident.

4. **Fantasy Imaging** (optional)

    a. Begin with a "known noun" image and interact to create fanciful, humorous images.
    b. Encourage student to create own fantasy images.

5. Group Instruction:
Apply this step to small groups of 3 to 5 students. Give one word to be described by all individuals in the group. Set the task as: *All students will help create one composite image, not separate images.* Each student will take a turn visualizing and verbalizing different aspects of the word to the group. The teacher will question, choose individuals to go through 3 or 4 structure words at a time, visualize, and summarize the composite image.

Chapter 6

Single Sentence Imaging

By now the student is able to visualize and verbalize given pictures and isolated words and the stimulation is wending its way toward building parts into a whole. The isolated word and this *single sentence* level establish visualizing and verbalizing for the "part" that will eventually construct the gestalt. Here the student will visualize and verbalize an isolated sentence. This is in preparation for the next step of *sentence by sentence imaging.*

Having said that, I often don't include this single sentence step! Many students can be moved from word imaging directly into sentence by sentence imaging. However, there are young or severely dysfunctional students who will need to move in small increments of language—a word, a phrase, a sentence—one step at a time. This level is for them.

The following lesson demonstrates how to have the student visualize the parts of a sentence—the words—and construct a sentence gestalt. Begin the step by overlapping from a known noun to a sentence. Use the noun just imaged and extend it to a sentence. The following lesson continues with Linda who has just visualized and verbalized the known noun—*cat*.

---

sample lesson 8: Single Sentence Imaging

Nanci: "We have been visualizing and verbalizing single words and now we will put those words together to form a sentence. A sentence is a thought, a concept. I'll read you the sentence and you visualize then verbalize it back to me.

The cat is under the chair.

Use the cat you just visualized. What do you see?"

Linda: "I see a cat under a chair."

Nanci: **"Those were the words I said, but tell me more about your image. I know to see the cat under a chair, but I don't know what kind of chair...a lawn chair outside, a wooden chair in the kitchen?"**

Note: It is critical to interact like this so the student will begin to refine both the visualization and the verbalization. It is very common for an individual with language difficulty to restate the words rather than visualize. Be alert to paraphrasing and don't assume imagery.

Linda: **"It's that striped cat I described earlier only now its under a chair in the kitchen."**

Nanci: **"Good. What do you see for the chair and the kitchen. Give me more details and background information. What the cat is doing under the chair...sleeping, drinking, eating, scratching..."**

The lesson continued with Linda responding to the above stimulation. I included fantasy imagery to lighten the session and still stimulate imagery.

Since I often omit this step entirely, only use and practice it based on need. Start with an overlap from a known noun and extend to simple and silly sentences. For example, present a simple sentence for detail imagery, hold a part of that image, and then modify some of the sentence to be silly.

1. The kitten looked in the mirror.
    The kitten looked in the mirror, jumped at itself, hissed, and ran way.

2. The circus clown stood up.
    The circus clown stood up, honked his big red nose, and did a somersault in the air.

3. The baby laughed.
    The baby laughed and put his hand in the birthday cake.

Underlining Image Words

After the student has visualized and verbalized receptively in simple sentences, have her read a simple sentence aloud and underline the image words. Diagnostically, you must have the student read aloud to be certain of accurate decoding. Obviously inaccurate decoding interferes with accurate imagery. Silent reading and V/V will be introduced later.

sample lesson 9: Underlining Image Words

Nanci: **"Now, I want you to read the sentence aloud and underline words that create an image."**

The cat is in the tree.

The student should underline as follows:

The <u>cat</u> is <u>in</u> the <u>tree</u>.

The lesson would continue with V/V for *detailed imagery*.

Although it could be argued that more words in the above sentence could be underlined, it would defeat the purpose of this lesson as well as fatigue the student. Therefore, underline only the critical image words in the sentence. The "the" could have been underlined since we aren't reading about "a" cat, but "the" is not a critical image word. I did underline "in" since it was a simple sentence with few image words and the cat was "in" the tree, not "under" the tree, or "behind" the tree.

Usually nouns, verbs, adverbs, and adjectives are the image words in a sentence. However, don't discuss underlining in grammatical terms, such as "underline the verbs and nouns." It has been my experience that even high school and college students are often not sure about the basic parts of speech. *This lesson is teaching imagery, not grammar.*

For further reference on the underlining technique, read "The Mind's Eye," a program from a Title IV project in the public schools at Escondido, California. Reading comprehension scores showed extremely significant gains just by having students underline image words.

Practice Single Sentence Imaging

Most students won't require this step and can just move from word imaging to sentence by sentence imaging. However, it can be a very important prerequisite for students with severe language impairment.

The same criteria for practice applies:
- Approximately 80% accuracy.
- Fair confidence with the task.
- Overlap to the next step to keep energy and interest.

Summary of Single Sentence Imaging

step 4

Objective: The student will be able to visualize and verbalize a sentence.

1. Single sentence imaging

    a. Overlap from a *known noun* to create a simple sentence.

    b. The student images parts of a sentence—words—to construct a sentence gestalt.

    c. Include *detailed imagery*.

    d. Include fanciful images by constructing a simple + silly sentence.

2. Underlining image words

    a. Student underlines the image words while reading the sentence orally.

    b. Do not teach a grammar lesson.

Note: The single sentence imaging step is optional. This type of stimulation often only requires modest attention or may be omitted completely.

Chapter 7

Sentence by Sentence Imaging from Oral and Written Language

All the stimulation up to this point has simply been in preparation for this step of **sentence by sentence imaging.** The majority of the stimulation is directed here. *This step should never be omitted* or treated modestly, for it is now that parts will be brought together to form a gestalt. At the single sentence imaging level, the student imaged the parts—the words—and created the whole of the sentence. At this *sentence by sentence* level, the student images the parts—the sentences—and creates the whole of the paragraph. *Sentences are imaged and connected to form the gestalt of a paragraph.*

As discussed earlier, when individuals have difficulty with language comprehension, they usually get "parts" of what they read or hear. They may, for example, remember a date, a name, a town, etc., but they have difficulty putting the parts together to grasp the gestalt. An anecdote will help you visualize and internalize this problem of forming imaged gestalts.

I had an opportunity to work with a physician who had always experienced weakness in comprehending language. He specifically mentioned that he had difficulty comprehending material he read and usually had to read it more than once. His wife said that he also had difficulty grasping movies, specifically movies that had a "flashback."

Since he was only visiting our area, I had just a few hours to try some Visualizing and Verbalizing with him. Initially, he had difficulty getting strong images from known nouns. After a little practice, we proceeded to the sentence by sentence level. I chose a third-grade skill book with short, self-contained, high-imagery paragraphs. I read him the first sentence. After a short time, and questioning, he imaged the sentence. I read him the next sentence from the same paragraph. He imaged that sentence, but his second image was completely unrelated to his first image. He was visualizing but he visualized two parts and no whole! Experimenting, I read the next sentence to him and again he finally imaged, but he imaged something completely unrelated to the first two sentences. Although I had read him only three sentences from a third-grade paragraph, he couldn't easily summarize the content. He told me a few parts but he had no gestalt. He could not tell me the main idea nor give me a cohesive summary of the material.

I continued to experiment by reading him an entire paragraph without interruptions. Again, he was unable to summarize the content. He gave me a few bits of information. I then had him read a paragraph to himself. He responded the same—parts and no gestalt.

His experience is not an isolated incident and he is not ignorant, dull, nor apathetic. He exhibited the same pattern that has emerged with all individuals who have this language comprehension weakness. Individuals of all ages, from all different backgrounds, share the common trait of perceiving parts but not gestalts. *It is therefore critical in* **sentence by sentence imaging** *that the sentence images build on one another to form a gestalt.*

The lessons begin receptively in order to remove decoding as a possible interference and stimulate oral language comprehension—auditory comprehension. Read aloud one sentence at a time. Have the student place a three-inch colored square on the table and visualize and verbalize the sentence back. The colored square simply anchors the sentence image—the parts. Require detailed imagery for the first sentence by using the structure words. The student will build one image onto the other, creating an imaged gestalt by the end of the paragraph. Two new steps are added to this level: a *Picture Summary* and *Word Summary*. Once the paragraph is completed, she gives a picture summary by verbally describing her images. She touches each colored square that has been placed for each sentence and says, *"Here I saw...."* Once the picture summary is completed, she gives a generalized verbal summary of the content in her own words. This paraphrasing is the word summary, using images for reference.

The Sentence by Sentence Steps

1. The teacher reads a sentence to the student.

2. The teacher questions with choice and contrast, *monitoring* the importance of questioning to the gestalt. Question to the main character or concept first, then outward like the structure words.

3. The student visualizes and verbalizes the sentence, placing a colored square to anchor the sentence image.

4. The student checks through the structure words to develop a detailed gestalt for only the **first** sentence.

5. The teacher reads the next sentence to the student, who then visualizes and verbalizes the sentence, placing another colored square.

6. The paragraph is completed, sentence by sentence.

7. The student touches each square and gives a *picture summary* by verbally describing the images created for each square.

8. The teacher collects the squares and the student gives a *word summary* by verbally summarizing the entire paragraph.

A picture summary describes images and a word summary paraphrases.

The student continues to be aware that her words will create images for you. This forces her to clarify and be specific with oral language expression. The lesson continues with Linda—her hair still greenish.

---

sample lesson 10: Sentence-by-Sentence Imaging

We are using a paragraph from the Richard Boning, *Specific Skills Series*. The text is:

> **Some spiders go fishing when they get hungry. The fisher spider climbs down plant stems into the water. The spider injects its powerful poison into the fish and drags it up on land, where it is eaten.**

Nanci: **"We are now going to visualize and verbalize a whole paragraph but we will do it sentence by sentence...and we will build one sentence image onto the other rather than having a bunch of separate images. We will use a colored square for each sentence image...and we will connect our images like this.** (I place 3 x 3 inch different colored squares, of paper or felt, in a vertical line, right next to one another.)

We want to make our images connect rather than having an image here, and another one here, and another one here." (I scatter colored squares around the table as I speak, to illustrate disconnected images).

Note: The colored squares are used to anchor the imaged parts.

Nanci: **"I'll read the first sentence to you: Some spiders go fishing when they get hungry.** *What do those words make you picture?* **When you get an image, choose a colored square and put it down in front of you."**

Linda: **"Some spiders go fishing when they are hungry."** (Linda places a colored square.)

95

Note: This is a very common response. Linda is paraphrasing. She just restated the words read to her. It is highly probable that she doesn't have a vivid image. She might just say back the words for each sentence and at the end of the paragraph be able to give only a few "parts" of the paragraph but no gestalt. It is also very common for her to just read words that go in one ear and out the other...with no connection. The problem may begin with dysfunction in imaging and then become habit.

Nanci: "Those were the words I read, but what images did those words give you? Let me read it to you again. Relax, and then let those words turn into pictures in your brain: **Some spiders go fishing when they get hungry.** "

Linda: "I see a spider who is fishing."

Nanci: "That is better. Now help me know what you're seeing for the spider. What size is the spider, where he is, even make a funny image?"

Linda: "It is a...tarantula spider, he is sitting in a lawn chair with a fishing pole, down by the river!"

Nanci: "That is a great picture! I can just see him...mine has on sunglasses! You did a good job of connecting to most of the sentence. Give me some details about the spider. Think about the structure words—how big, what color, what does the lawn chair look like?"

Linda: "He is about this big (gesturing about three inches).... He is brownish black with sunglasses on."

Nanci: "What is he sitting on? Give me some more details about the background."

Linda: "He is laying, sort of, on a yellow lawn chair, next to a river, with a fishing pole in his hand. The river is right in front of him. He's on the bank."

We discussed the river a little more—not so much as to deviate from the main idea, just to be sure she had a detailed image.

Nanci: "Let me read the sentence to you again because there is one more thing you need to see in this sentence: **Some spiders go fishing when they get hungry.**"

Linda: "Oh...hungry. I see him rubbing his tummy (gesturing) and he has a fishing hat on with those little hooks and things on it."

Nanci: "Great!   Now let's check through the structure words for this first sentence—just to be sure we have all the details."

We checked through each structure word and developed a detailed gestalt for the first sentence.

Nanci: "Good. I'll read you the next sentence. Remember the next image will be connected to this one...not something separate...so when we are through we will have a complete movie in our heads. We might have to change some parts of our image because do you think spiders can really fish with a fishing pole?"

Linda: "No. But that helps me to remember my image and it is fun."

Nanci: "Right. Here is the next sentence: **The fisher spider climbs down plant stems into the water.** What do those words make you picture? Now we have to change the first picture a little, but you can keep the same general setting and the same spider."

Linda: "I see my spider getting into the water on a plant."

Nanci: "Place the second colored square for this sentence, and show me what you see...Use your hands."

Linda places the square but appears confused and says something about a plant and water with the spider falling into the water. It was obvious that she was just paraphrasing. We pursue images.

Nanci: "Let me read it to you again and see if your image gets better: **The fisher spider climbs down plant stems.**"

Linda: "I see a plant in the water and the spider is climbing down it."

Nanci: "What does the plant look like? What color, what size do you picture? What part of the plant is the spider climbing down? Show me with your hands."

Linda: "The plant is about this tall...and is green. The spider is climbing down it... like this."

Nanci: "That is a lot clearer. So the sentence says: **The fisher spider climbs down plant stems into the water.** What did you see the spider do when he got down the plant stem?"

Linda: "He took off his hat and jumped into the water. Well, actually, his hat fell off as he was going down the stem!"

Nanci: "Great! Let me read some more so we can find out how this spider catches the fish if he doesn't use a fishing pole. **The spider injects its powerful poison into the fish and drags it up on land, where it is then eaten.** What do those words make you picture?"

I have her place the third colored square as she begins to describe her image.

Note: Note that I use the question, *"What do those words make you picture"* after I read the stimulus. A very important question; use it often.

Linda: "Hmmmm, I see him with big things coming out of his mouth. What do you call those...oh, I remember, fangs. I see these fangs coming out of his mouth and he shoots some stuff at the fish. Then he takes the fish out and...I don't know."

Nanci: "You did a good job of imaging the first part about the spider and his fangs. What do you see coming out of the spider's mouth? You just said stuff."

Linda: "I don't know...some poison stuff."

Nanci: "When you say the word 'poison' I get a better picture in my brain of what the stuff was. What color do you see?"

Linda: "White."

Nanci: "Good. I'll read it again and let's see what happens after he shoots the fish with the white poison: **The spider injects its powerful poison into the fish and drags it up on land, where it is eaten.**"

Linda: "I see him taking the fish to the shore and then...ripping into it."

Nanci: "What did the fish look like? Was it big or little and how did you see him getting it out of the water...with a rope or what?"

Linda: "The fish is real big, like this (gesturing to the width of her arm span and laughing). I don't know how he got it out."

Nanci: "That is a fun image but do you really think a spider could kill and haul a big fish out of the water? Show me again how big your spider was...and the fish is this big...will the spider be able to move it?"

98

Linda: "No. I'll make it a little fish...like a blue gill which is this big (gesturing about six inches)."

Nanci: "That is better. Let me show you how big my fish was (gesturing the size of a little goldfish). I visualized a little fish so I could imagine that the spider got it out of the water. Try to visualize that."

Note: I modeled and imposed my image into her imaged gestalt.

Linda: "Yeah, that's better. Just a little fish, like this...."

Nanci: "How did the spider get the fish out of the water? That is still pretty unusual...to think of a spider getting a fish out of the water. The sentence said: **and drags it up on land, where it is eaten.** What is the 'it' in this sentence?"

Linda: "Oh, I see...(begins to laugh)...I see him put a big net around the fish and then he pulls it to the land."

Nanci: "Great! Then what does he do?"

Linda: "He begins to tear into it with his big teeth! And then he goes back in the water after his hat!"

Nanci: "Excellent imaging and connecting your images. The whole story had the same spider and the same river. Now, you have three colored squares out here for those images. Give me a picture summary...which tells me what you pictured for each square. All you have to tell me is the image you had for that square and it doesn't have to be with as much detail."

Beginning a picture summary:

Linda proceeded to retell her image for each square (sentence). She touched each one and began her sentence with *"Here I saw."*

Linda: Pointing to square #1:
"Here I saw a brownish/black spider, sitting on a lawn chair next to a river. He had on sunglasses and a hat and was rubbing his tummy."

Pointing to square #2:

"Here I saw the spider climbing down a green plant, and jumping into the water."

Pointing to square #3:

"Here I saw the spider, with big fangs, shoot poison into this little gold fish. Then he put a net around the fish and pulled it to the bank and tore into it."

Note: If Linda paused long enough to indicate she needed a prompt—I would have given her a picture-cue to help her retrieve her sentence image.

Beginning a word summary

Nanci: **"Great. Now give me a word summary, using your images to help retell the story. We'll take the squares away...just tell me what this was about."**

Linda: **"I saw a spider about this big."**

Nanci: **"Wait, that would be a picture summary. When you give a word summary, you just tell me the story over again. For instance, pretend I just walked in the room and said, Hi Linda. What did you hear about today?"**

Linda: **"I heard about a spider...he lives by a river and he...(eyes up indicating imaging)...climbs down a plant in the water and shoots poison at a fish and then takes the fish back to shore and eats it."**

Nanci: **"Perfect...and you didn't say anything about his hat and sunglasses and yellow chair...because they were only our images and weren't in the actual story."**

These elements should be noted at the sentence by sentence level.

1. **Begin receptively to develop oral language comprehension**
    Begin to develop oral language comprehension prior to developing written language comprehension. You read to the student and remove decoding as a possible interference in the imaging process.

2. **Extend to written language comprehension**
    As the student acquires some proficiency with receptive sentence by sentence imaging, begin to have her read each sentence aloud to develop written language comprehension. Work all comprehension processes simultaneously: receptive, oral reading, and silent reading.

3. **Detailed imagery for the initial sentence**
It is important to develop detailed imagery in the early stages of the sentence by sentence level and also develop a gestalt, not separate images. The images must be linked to one another. It is very helpful to establish a strong image for the initial sentence because short paragraphs are often written with the topic sentence, the main idea, as the first sentence. Consequently establishing a detailed image for it will assist the student in creating a gestalt.

4. **Connecting images from sentence to sentence**
Occasionally, a paragraph will have a second sentence that deviates from the first sentence. However, there is usually a way to connect the first image with the second image. For example, in one of the Boning Specific Skills books there is a paragraph that starts like this: *Enemies may pass the snowshoe rabbit without even seeing it.* This usually creates an image of a white rabbit in a snow area and an enemy, such as a fox or wolf, walking by without noticing the rabbit. The next sentence has a moderate deviation: *Although brown in summer, it puts on a coat of white in winter and becomes almost impossible to see.* If we image the rabbit as "brown in the summer," we do not need to have a completely different picture. We can keep the same rabbit and the same background but just change the season and color of the rabbit.

The same connection can be made with almost every paragraph you choose. On the occasions when the first two sentences turn out to be completely unrelated, which is rare, I simply solve the problem by choosing another paragraph! This is appropriate at the sentence by sentence level which is a developmental stage rather than a refinement stage. However, the problem can be completely prevented by the teacher scanning the paragraphs prior to "visualizing and verbalizing" them.

5. **Use of the structure words**
Use the *structure words* to establish that important detailed image for only the first sentence. However, it is only necessary to check through the structure words in the initial lessons of the sentence by sentence level. Later, the student will be including all the details automatically.

Remember to use the structure words only for the first sentence/image. If the structure words were used for each sentence, the lesson would become lengthy and tedious, with no joy or energy.

6. **Placing a colored square for each sentence**
The student will place a colored square for each sentence as a means of anchoring images and providing a structure from which to think. I usually place the squares *vertically* on the table, from top to bottom, just like I read a paragraph. Some teachers/tutors have chosen to place them from left to right.

Any method of placing will achieve the purpose of anchoring images, as long as the relevancy of the session is not impeded.

The colored squares are 3" x 3" squares of felt or paper. They are different colors, although color has nothing to do with the image represented. I have not found it useful to use certain colors, shapes, or objects to anchor sentence images. The purpose of the colored square is not to cue an image but to act as an anchor for each "part."

7. **Picture summary**

The summary of the paragraph begins with a *picture summary*. The student points to a colored square and sequentially describes her picture for that particular square. The verbalization should begin with the phrase, "Here I saw..." It is important to include this step at the sentence by sentence level to be certain that she is visualizing and not paraphrasing. The process is effective only if visualization is stimulated. At this level, picture summaries are relevant in terms of imagery and sequential reverbalization.

8. **Word summary**

A *word summary* requires the individual to verbally summarize the paragraph using images to support the verbalization. It is often more difficult than a picture summary. Picture summaries let the student just describe her images. Since describing images was developed prior to the sentence by sentence level, by now it is fairly easy for her. Word summaries use images for support but require verbal generalizing.

Here are some ways to help the student initiate a word summary:

a. It is helpful to initiate a word summary with action and fun. I often get up from my chair, walk out, and then walk in again. I pretend to just be arriving on the scene, having never before heard the story. This often effectively stimulates a word summary because it places the student in a real situation. Pretending not to have heard the story before means that the student must tell you everything. The "play" aspect of the technique contributes to reducing the individuals' stress regarding verbalizing and just generally lightens the oh-so-serious atmosphere of learning.

b. In the initial word summary lessons, it is often necessary to initiate the verbal summary for the student. For example, "This story was about a spider that..." or begin with a partial statement, "The fisher spider catches...."

c. It is sometimes necessary to redirect the student from a picture summary to a word summary. In the initial sessions of giving a word summary, the

102

student is very likely to retell just images for squares, thus giving a picture summary. She will need help modifying the verbalization from talking about the images to telling a general summary. Discuss the difference between a picture summary—where all the fantasy images can be recalled —and a word summary—where the images are used for recalling concepts but are not stated verbally.

d. A student may struggle through a word summary until thoughts become disassembled and lack cohesiveness and fluency. It is then helpful either to have the student retell the summary, which probably will improve fluency, or to model the retelling.

9. **Questioning critical to imagery**
Follow each stimulus with: *"What do those words make you picture?"*

Use an inquiry technique. Notice that I did not let Linda just say the words back, paraphrase. It is important to be alert to paraphrasing by the student and not assume she is imaging just because *you* are imaging. It only takes a few minutes to ask some questions that will let you know if she is really imaging and those same questions will *create* images.

Always question to the gestalt. I have observed teachers struggle while learning to question. They often question for images but get lost in detail and minutia, and don't develop an imaged gestalt.

10. **Monitor amount of verbalizing from teacher**
Often students with weak language processing are not very verbal. They do not express themselves easily and therefore may not be talkative. This presents you with a situation to monitor closely. Are you doing all the talking and assuming the student is "getting it?"

11. **Automaticity with imaging is the goal**
The goal is for the student to image automatically **as** she reads or receives language. Begin to note if she is reacting and interacting with language by moving eyes up, defocusing, or reacting emotionally. A college student told me he began to image after a few weeks, but the "big difference came when I could see a movie...when it all come together automatically."

12. **Begin with low-level material**
Sentence by sentence imaging should always begin in low-level material and stay there until the imaging has reached a fair level of automaticity. I begin with third-grade material since the paragraphs are high imagery and short, thus reducing the amount of content necessary to create the gestalt. If your student is

below third-grade, begin with low-level paragraphs at the primer or first-grade level. Modify these paragraphs to add more interest and images.

13. How to correct an erroneous image
If the individual gives you an erroneous image or leaves something out, reread the sentence to her. Preface that with, "Let me reread this to you and see if you want to add or change anything." You may even need to call attention to the specific image to be visualized. For example, if the student visualized "a cat in the woods" but the language indicated "a cat in the city," ask the student to listen and check for where the cat should be visualized.

14. Correcting a picture summary
Occasionally, the student will lose the image for a specific colored square. When this happens, simply cue a part of the image back for the student. For example, "This square is where you saw the red...." Usually the student will immediately retrieve the image and respond with, "Oh, that's right, here I saw...."

15. Correcting a word summary
The student may begin a word summary that doesn't include enough detail. At that point, you can use images to help the student monitor the verbalization. For example, if the student says, "This was about how birds get destroyed," you can reply, "Your words make me picture birds being destroyed by a laser beam, or elephants, or giant cats, or...." The purpose is to illustrate again that the words create images. This stimulation encourages the student to monitor expressive language so as to be specific and is excellent preparation for paragraph writing.

16. Grade level of material
Initially use lower grade level material—such as third grade—despite the age of the student. Obviously, if the student is younger than third grade, use low-level material appropriate for that student. As proficiency develops for her in sentence by sentence processing, increase the difficulty of the paragraphs. For example, as Linda becomes more apt at visualizing and verbalizing, I will move her from third to fourth grade, and so on, until I have her processing automatically, sentence by sentence at or *above* her grade level.

17. Student reads orally and silently
Initially you will read each sentence to the student. As the stimulation progresses, begin to have the student read each sentence aloud. It is very important to have her read since she will be applying this to her written work and you won't be available to read all material aloud. Eventually begin to have her read each sentence silently, continuing the same procedure of visualizing and verbalizing each sentence. Simultaneously continue stimulation for oral

language comprehension, oral reading comprehension, and silent reading comprehension.

18. Content

The content to be visualized and verbalized is not really relevant, except it should be a high-imagery, self-contained, short paragraph. Remember you are not teaching content. You are teaching *process*.

Practice Sentence by Sentence

Sentence by sentence visualizing and verbalizing is truly the heart of the V/V process. This level develops the individuals' ability to create imaged gestalts and give verbal summaries. Because of its critical relationship to the success of the rest of the V/V process, this level must be practiced vigorously. The goal is for the student to *automatically* visualize a gestalt from the imaged parts and give both a picture and word summary. Adhere to a rigid practice plan. This level cannot be practiced too much for it is at this step that the student begins to visualize and verbalize the gestalt. The teacher verbalized the gestalt in all previous steps. Increase the difficulty of the material and continue practicing. Vary the tasks to keep lesson energy and joy.

Sentence by Sentence

1. Nanci reads a sentence to Linda.

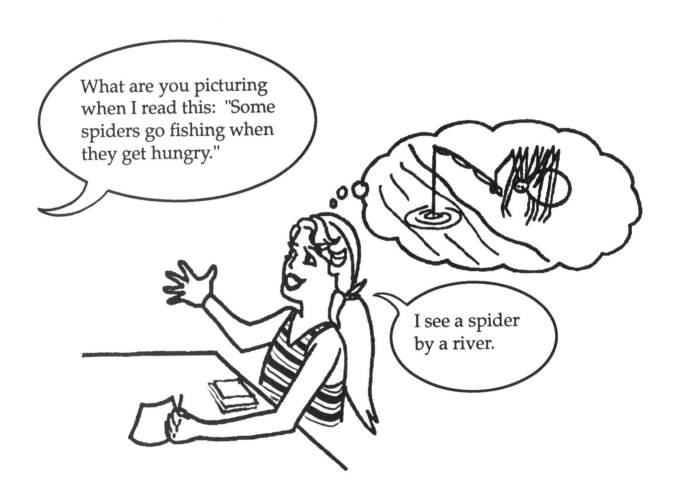

2. Nanci questions to develop detailed imagery.

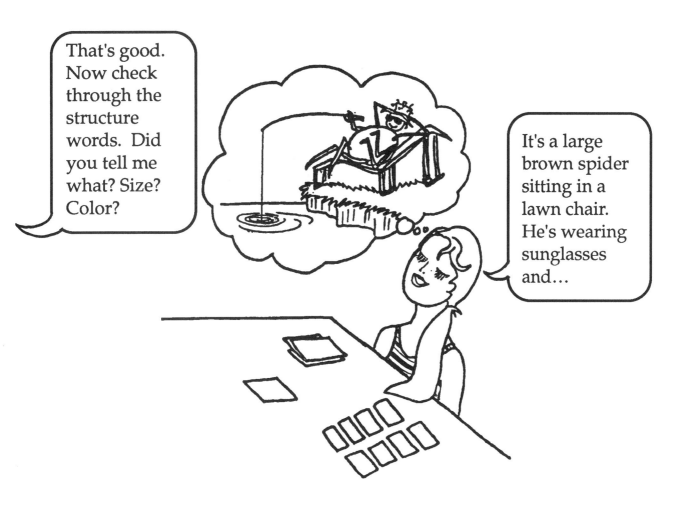

3. Linda gives a "picture summary."

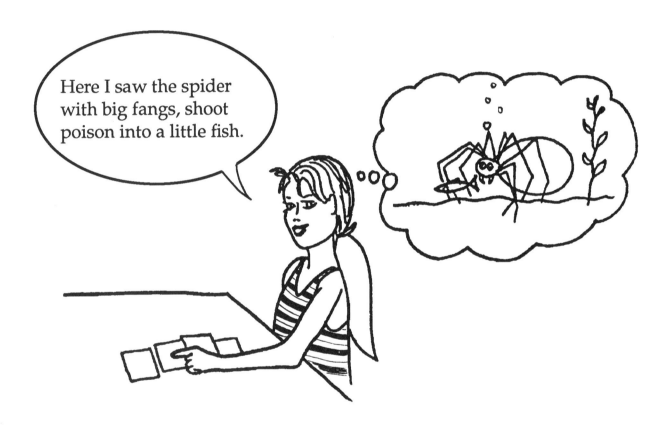

4. Linda gives a "word summary."

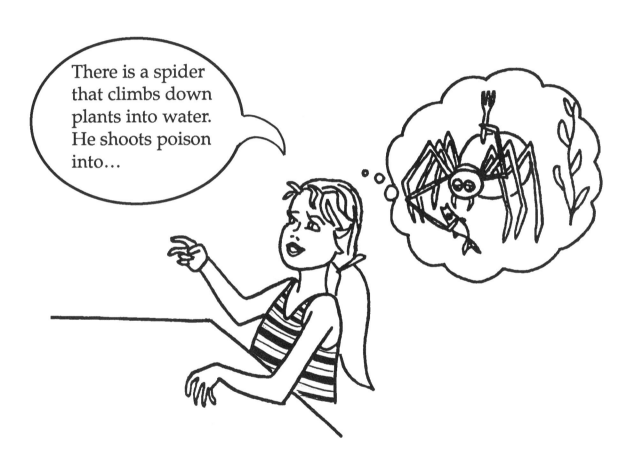

Summary of Sentence by Sentence Imaging

step 5

Objective: The student will image a paragraph gestalt by visualizing and verbalizing each sentence of a paragraph, then verbalizing a picture summary and word summary.

1. The student images each sentence to create a paragraph gestalt.

2. The teacher interacts by questioning to develop an imaged gestalt.

3. The structure words are checked through for the first sentence to develop detailed imagery for topic sentence.

4. The student gives a *picture summary*—touches each felt and says: "Here I saw... "

5. The student gives a *word summary*—a verbal summary that uses images to formulate generalizations.

6. The sentence images build on one another rather than separate parts.

7. Question or comment with choice and contrast to create images for the student. Follow each sentence stimulus with: "What do those words make you picture?"

8. Be alert to paraphrasing, rather than imaging.

9. Begin receptively—you read each sentence to the student. Later the student will read each sentence orally or silently, continuing the same general technique of giving a picture and word summary.

10. Begin to diagnose for automatic imaging.

11. Initially, use low-level material, despite age or grade level. Increase the paragraph difficulty as the student acquires proficiency.

12. Present material in all three modes:
    a. You read each sentence to the student (receptive)
    b. Student reads each sentence aloud (expressive)
    c. Student reads each sentence to self (same procedure of placing colored square and verbalizing images)

13. Correct picture summaries by cuing the student with a part of the image.

14. Correct word summaries by using the phrase: "Your words made me picture..." Spice up an erroneous image to encourage the student to be specific with the verbalization.

15. Reread a sentence to clarify a specific image.

16. *Sentence by sentence level is critical—practice vigorously.*

17. **Group Instruction:**
    Consider the small group—3 to 5 students—a collective individual. All students participate in the same paragraph. Choose a different student to: 1) visualize and verbalize each sentence, 2) check through the structure words on first sentence, 3) verbalize the picture summary, and 4) verbalize the word summary.

Chapter 8

Sentence by Sentence
Higher Order Thinking Skills

The sentence by sentence sessions usually continue for weeks or months and this next step extends it into higher order thinking skills, (HOTS). *It is critical to include this sentence by sentence with higher order thinking skills step.*

The taxonomy of comprehension skills includes the following:

- Locating and Remembering (recalling facts)
- Getting the Main Idea
- Inferring
- Drawing Conclusions
- Predicting/Extending
- Evaluating

It is believed that the easiest comprehension skill is to "locate and remember" details of information. Experience with the V/V process confirms that premise. Individuals with weak imagery and comprehension skills are often able to recall a few facts of what they have read or heard. However, they have no base from which to process the main idea, make an inference, draw a conclusion or make a general summary. Their difficulty constructing an imaged gestalt interferes with their higher order thinking skills, reasoning, and analytical thinking.

The sentence by sentence level developed the imaged gestalt from which individuals can reason. As discussed above, if individuals have only a few details in mind, they cannot put together the main idea of the information from either oral or written language. The same premise is valid for the other levels of comprehension skills. Skills such as inferring, drawing conclusions, predicting, and evaluating all require a "whole" from which to process. If individuals are primarily processing details, they will make erroneous assumptions, generalizations, summaries, conclusions, predictions, and evaluations. *The ability to process the gestalt of information is the foundation for higher level comprehension and thinking skills.*

115

Sentence by sentence lessons are the core of the V/V process and now extend to *developing* interpretive comprehension and thinking skills. An actual lesson with a boy named Jerry will help demonstrate the process. Jerry is a good-looking boy with dark-blond hair, a round face, and a shy affect. He usually wears a military fatigue cap. He is 11 years old and has just completed sixth grade. He has a receptive vocabulary of a 14-year-old, word recognition skills at the ninth-grade level, and word attack skills at the twelfth-grade level. However, even with these strengths, his reading comprehension is unstable at the third-grade level. He is struggling in school and his mother described him as quiet and unable to express himself well. She stated, "When Jerry talks, it is fragmented. He usually tells the last first. We are all frustrated with him." His parents, both school teachers, are very concerned. He has a reading problem, but not a decoding problem. His school, like most others, gives priority to the children with decoding problems. Therefore, Jerry does not qualify for special reading classes. Both his parents and teachers are confused and concerned and have wondered if Jerry's problem is really just a lack of motivation. This is Jerry's first lesson at this level. We have not specifically applied sentence by sentence to higher order thinking yet.

sample lesson 11: Sentence by Sentence Imaging for HOTS

We continue to use the Richard Boning, *Specific Skills Series*. The text is:

> **Those who watch birds have seen them take dust baths. They flutter around dipping in the dust like children playing in the bathtub. Birds do this for a reason and that is that they try to get rid of the little bugs that are in their feathers.**

Nanci: "I will read a sentence to you and you'll visualize it as you have been...we'll place a colored square for each image. Here we go. **Those who watch birds have seen them take dust baths.** What do those words make you picture?"

Jerry: "It's like a blackbird...and he's like down on a farm that has dried out. The rain hasn't come on that farm in a long time. The bird is just like in the pig pen, rolling in the dust."

Nanci: "Good. Now give more details. What do you picture for the bird and the background?"

Note: Because Jerry is a little move advanced, I tried asking him an open-ended question rather than giving him choices. He proceeded to give a little

116

more detail. We interacted but because his images still appeared to be vague I decided to have him reverbalize through the structure words.

Nanci: **"OK. Let's go through the structure words and see if you have given me a lot of details on this first sentence."**

Jerry: **"Hmmm...."**

Nanci: (Pointing to the structure word cards on the table) **"Did you tell me *what* it was?"**

Jerry: **"Uh-huh."**

Nanci: **"Ok...just check through the cards and see if you want to tell me anything more. You told me you saw a blackbird."**

Jerry: **"Uh-huh...and I told you it was on the farm. I didn't tell you how big it was."**

Nanci: **"Right. Tell me a little more about what you see for the blackbird."**

Jerry: **"The blackbird is about that big (gesturing)."**

Nanci: **"OK."**

Jerry: **"And...he's rolling around in the dust...and walking around in the dust."**

Nanci: **"OK. You have told me about the color and the shape. Can you tell me some background? You said on the farm, but as we zero right in on the bird, let's get a really good picture of what it looks like around him. We can see dust and what else?"**

Jerry: **"Pigs are around him...and horses."**

Nanci: **"Oh pigs, I forgot that you said pigs. Where shall I see the pigs?"**

Jerry: **"Trying to get in as much mud as they can."**

Nanci: **"So, if the pigs are trying to get in the mud, is the bird by the pigs? Is he trying to get in the mud too?"**

Jerry: **"No. He's in the dust."**

Nanci: "OK. Do you see fences or are the pigs just walking around? I don't know what you really see."

Jerry: "They are looking for mud somewhere and trying to keep in the shade too."

Note: I have to be careful not to question his images for pigs or I will lose the gestalt of this paragraph.

Nanci: "OK. So...where is the bird in all this?"

Jerry: "The pigs are over here (gesturing to a place on the table), trying to get mud and then the birds are over here trying to get dust...and the pen goes like this...."

Nanci: "OK...so they are in a pen. I didn't know you saw that. What do you see for the time of day? Like this structure word says *when*... Do you I see morning or night?"

Jerry: "Afternoon. It's in the afternoon."

Note: Because it is difficult to visualize "afternoon," it is likely that he just gave me a time but did not image anything. Therefore, I question a little further to try to stimulate some imagery.

Nanci: "Hot or cold? Sunny or cloudy? Give me some idea of what you see for that."

Jerry: "Hot! Hot and sunny."

Nanci: "And *movement*...you told me that he was doing what?"

Jerry: "Rolling around and walking around."

Nanci: "Rolling around! It's a strange thing to think of a bird rolling around. Is he rolling over and over?"

Jerry: "Sort of like that (gesturing)."

Nanci: "Is he doing anything with his feet or feathers or wings?"

Jerry: "Uh-huh. He's using them to scratch the dust."

Nanci: **"What do you see him doing with his wings? I have a picture of him doing something with his wings and I wonder if you do."**

Jerry: **"He's just flopping them up (gesturing)."**

Nanci: **"Yes, that's what I saw him doing. "**

Jerry: **"Uh-huh...and they are making a lot of dust."**

Note: Are you noticing how little verbalization is coming from Jerry? He is responding to my image-making questions but he is not "visualizing and verbalizing" well on his own. His affect is flat, he doesn't respond well to humor, and he obviously still has difficulty visualizing and verbalizing automatically.

Nanci: **"That's what I saw too...the dust sort of swirling around the bird. This next structure word is *mood*."**

Jerry: (Interrupting) **"I saw three birds."**

Nanci: **"Oh! I thought you said you only pictured one blackbird. OK...now your words make me picture three blackbirds. I can just add a few to my original picture. What do you see for *mood*?"**

Jerry: **"They're happy."**

Nanci: We check through the remaining structure words and continue. **"All right...let's add on to it then. The next sentence is: They flutter about dipping in the dust like children playing in the bathtub. Our first picture was so good that we got almost all of that."**

Jerry: (Placing second colored square)... **"What is flutter?"**

Nanci: **"Good question. Flutter is like this (gesturing)... My fingers are fluttering here...like kicking when you are swimming."**

Jerry: **"Oh yeah...then their wings are fluttering. So, I picture that they are standing there and their wings are out like this and they are making a lot of dust with their wings."**

Nanci: **"Yes. Let's see if you got all of it. It says They flutter about dipping in the dust like children playing in the bathtub. Do you want to add or change anything to your picture?"**

119

Jerry: **"Yeah, they put their head under the dust and they go...**(he moves his head like it is dipping up and down in the dust).**"**

Nanci: Both grinning at the pictures they are getting.... **"Right, when it says: like children playing in the bathtub...do those words make you picture anything?"**

Jerry: "Uh-huh...(smiling)...they are like splashing around."

Nanci: "Yes...like children splashing in a bathtub...we won't get too much detail for that."

Note: I chose not to pursue a detailed image of the children in the bathtub—just as I didn't pursue detailed images for the pigs in the first sentence. Both pursuits would have lengthened the lesson and were not relevant to the gestalt.

Nanci: **"Let's do the last sentence: Birds do this for a reason and that is that they try to get rid of the little bugs that are in their feathers. What do those words make you picture?"** (I hand Jerry the third colored square.)

Jerry: **"Well, they are flapping their wings trying to get the bugs out of their wings."**

Note: Now there is some doubt as to whether Jerry is paraphrasing or imaging. Note how I proceed.

Nanci: **"How can you see that part...them trying to get the bugs out?"**

Jerry: **"They are picking at their wings and things."**

Nanci: **"Good. Also, we had to add something to our picture that we didn't have before. We had birds but now we had to add something else. Do you know what it was?"**

Jerry: **"Them trying to get bugs out of their wings."**

Nanci: **"Bugs! We had to add bugs to it. In order to picture that sentence you had to add bugs to your birds. Where do you see the bugs?"**

Jerry: **"Going in and out of their feathers trying to keep on!"**

Nanci: "Yes...I can get in close now with my picture and I can see the birds right here...(gesturing)...and I can see their feathers and see little bugs hopping around."

Note: I modeled images for him which helped him visualize...note his next response.

Jerry: Grinning... "Little feather lice."

Nanci: "Exactly. In order to remember that part of the story, you would have to picture the bugs. You don't want to just say words back...you have to actually picture the bugs."

Beginning a picture summary:

Nanci: "Well, you have done a very good job. We have three squares out here for your images. Let's see if you can give me a picture summary. Remember to begin with *here I saw ....*"

Jerry: Touching the first square... "Here I saw the birds rolling around in the dust."

Nanci: "Yes...can you give me a little bit more detail for it?"

Jerry: "Well... see blackbirds walking around, with pigs nearby trying to find mud, and they were just making a lot of dust."

Nanci: "OK...what do you picture for this one?" (Touching second colored square).

Jerry: No response.

Nanci: (cuing back the image)... "We sort of came in closer on our birds on this one."

Jerry: "Ummm...here I saw they were putting their heads under the dust and shaking it off and they were making a lot of dust with their wings."

Nanci: "Yes. That one is where we saw them doing the fluttering...you showed me that movement...and the last picture that we had."

Jerry: Touching the third square... "Here I saw...they are trying to get bugs out of their feathers."

Nanci: "Yes...what is on the birds now and what do you see them doing?"

Jerry: "I see little bugs...and birds trying to get as much dust on themselves as they can and then shaking them off."

Beginning a word summary:

Nanci: "That was a good picture summary. Now, give me a word summary. Pretend I just walked in the room and said to you, what did you hear today Jerry?"

Jerry: A long pause, slight sigh...and finally... "I read about birds taking a dust bath...."

Nanci: "OK...tell me all of it. Use the pictures you have in your head to reconstruct the story for me."

Jerry: More pause... "Blackbirds on a farm...in a dust pile. They flap their wings and dip in the dust, putting their head in the dust and shaking it off. They were trying to get bugs out of their feathers."

Nanci: "That was a good word summary. You didn't have to tell me it was blackbirds even though that was your picture. Did the author say it was just blackbirds that took a dust bath?"

Jerry: "No, it could be any birds, I guess."

Nanci: "Right. So you could just say 'birds,' or else we would think that it was only blackbirds that take dust baths."

Beginning to develop MAIN IDEA:

Nanci: "What was the main idea of that story? Now that we have that whole thing pictured...we can decide about the main thing this was trying to tell us."

Jerry: "The main thing?"

Nanci: "Yes...was it about how birds fly south...or how birds..."

Jerry: "No...it was about birds and dust baths."

Nanci: "Give me some more information. Just birds and dust baths?"

122

Jerry: "Birds take dust baths to try and get bugs out of their wings and feathers."

Nanci: "Exactly! That is exactly right. Now let me ask you another question...."

Beginning to develop INTERPRETIVE SKILLS:

Nanci: Inference: "Why do you think they take a dust bath and not a water bath?"

Jerry: "Because...because...the dust could pollute the air that the bugs breathe and that would make them get out."

We cough a little, and choke, like the bugs might cough and choke from the dust. I was impressed and somewhat surprised at the quality of Jerry's thinking. I had been considering a response based on how difficult it might be to locate shallow water to wash out the bugs!

We explored my thinking about water and I asked another inference question and then we drew a conclusion about the bathing procedures of birds. Interpretive questions are easily answered from an imaged gestalt.

How to ask HOTS questions

- An *inference* question is usually asking why.

- A question that asks the student to *draw a conclusion* usually begins with the statement, "from all this information we can conclude that..."

- A *predicting/extending* question usually asks the student to think of "what would happen next"...or "if...then we can predict that..."

- An *evaluative* question requires the student to evaluate the material based on his experience/information and these short paragraphs don't easily lend themselves to an evaluation. Therefore, I omit asking evaluative questions until the student is reading/receiving an entire page of information.

Analysis of sample lesson 11

Although the previous session appears lengthy in print, in practice the lesson lasted only 12 minutes. I chose to include this lesson because of the severity of Jerry's language processing problem. His reluctance and inability to verbalize required me to model and question with choice and contrast. It was a typical sample lesson at the sentence by sentence level that was extended to higher order thinking skills. Note the following:

1. **Begin receptively**

   As I stated earlier, it is important to begin receptively. I read to Jerry in order to keep the task focused on "visualizing and verbalizing" and not decoding. Inaccurate decoding interferes with imagery. Once students begin to demonstrate proficiency in visualizing and verbalizing receptively, then they should read orally and later read silently. I instructed Jerry's tutor to begin alternating the manner in which Jerry received the language for each paragraph. For example, she read, then he read aloud, and then he read silently. The lesson procedure is unchanged.

2. **Structure words**

   Structure words are optional. They may be used to develop detailed imagery for the first sentence; however, by now it is expected that students may automatically include details in their images.

3. **Picture summary and colored squares**

   Picture summaries continue at this sentence by sentence level for HOTS. The student places a square for each sentence as he reads the material and when the paragraph is completed *he touches each one* and verbalizes a picture summary by saying, "Here I saw...."

4. **Word summary**

   The student verbalizes a word summary by simply restating the information in his own words. Jerry wanted to include blackbirds, but the author didn't specify blackbirds, just birds. Nor did the author mention a farm and pigs, so Jerry's word summary had to omit those imagined details, though they had helped him image the language he read.

5. **Draw images?**

   Should the student be encouraged to draw his images? *Usually not*. Most individuals can image more effectively and efficiently than they can draw. The imagination is more apt than eye-hand coordination at creating elaborate, colorful, moving images.

6. **Main Idea**

   It is vital in the V/V process to develop higher level comprehension skills. Once the student can give accurate word summaries, it is fairly easy to teach the concept of main idea. Remember, the main idea of a paragraph can be grasped only if the individual has the gestalt of the material. Individuals who recall, or connect to, only details of the information will not be able to generalize to a main idea, nor any other higher level comprehension skills.

Although easily taught, the student will usually need practice learning how to analyze and state the main idea. He will frequently give a statement that is too broad rather than too narrow. Either way, it is very helpful to use the principle of contrast in stimulating his thought processes. Giving him contrasting images/thoughts from which to generate usually illustrates to him the need for clarification.

For example, Jerry gave a very general main idea statement when he said, "This was about birds." Using the principle of contrast, I can reply with, "Is it about birds eating worms, about birds standing on their heads, about birds making nests...?" This allows Jerry to see that he needs to provide information since his words didn't give me enough information to visualize. By giving feedback regarding the images that his words made me create, he began to monitor his verbalization.

When using the principle of contrast to stimulate, give choices that create powerful or interesting images. The purpose of the lesson is to develop language processing through imagery, so provide choices with flair. It is interesting to note that very frequently students with weak language processing also have very bland images with no color, no excitement, no imagination, no movement, and no creativity! You must prompt it with your choices.

Also, as with a word summary, it is often helpful to prompt the main idea sentence by initiating the sentence with a few beginning words that direct the student to the concept of the main idea. Or, you may even model a good or poor main idea.

7. **Inferring, predicting, concluding, evaluating**
Inferring, concluding, predicting and extending, and evaluating should be introduced at the sentence by sentence level. Once the student can give accurate word summaries and main idea statements, it is easy to begin asking an inference or prediction question. I usually begin with inference questions for a few sessions and extend to prediction questions, followed later by conclusion and occasionally evaluation questions. Inference questions are usually "why" questions and prediction questions are usually "What do you think would happen if..." questions. Asking a conclusion question simply means asking the individual to draw a conclusion by saying, "From all this information we can conclude that...."

An evaluation question is primarily asking the student to evaluate the information in terms of how he or she feels about it. As stated earlier, it is usually not necessary to do much with evaluation questions at the sentence by sentence level because the material is simple and short and doesn't lend itself to evaluation. Later in the V/V process, an entire page of material will be visualized and verbalized, which can be personally evaluated.

It is important to remember that the gestalt base is a prerequisite to these higher order thinking skills and if the student is still struggling with *word summaries*, then you should not begin these questions. He would have a limited framework from which to process the question.

Practice Sentence by Sentence Imaging HOTS

Sentence by sentence imaging for higher order thinking must be practiced until the student is processing the gestalt easily—evidenced by fluent, confident picture and word summaries—and is answering interpretive questions reasonably well. Keep in mind that interpretive questions were *introduced* at this level and will continue to be asked throughout the remaining V/V process. At the following levels of *Multiple Sentence Imaging* and *Whole Paragraph Imaging* there will be more *lesson energy* available for interpretive thinking because the student will be visualizing and verbalizing with more ease and confidence.

Increase the difficulty of the material as is appropriate. Do not stay in low level material. As the student develops visualizing and verbalizing skills, move slowly to more difficult levels. For example, move from third-grade to fourth-grade, but stay at the fourth grade level until a fair amount of confidence and skill is demonstrated, then move up another level.

Summary of Sentence by Sentence with HOTS

step 6

Objective: The student will be able to visualize and verbalize sentence-by-sentence, continuing to develop a paragraph gestalt, and *begin* to develop higher order thinking skills.

1. The student visualizes each sentence to create a paragraph gestalt, using colored squares.

2. The teacher interacts, *beginning* to ask open-ended questions rather than choice/contrast questions.

3. The structure words might be used for first sentence.

4. The student verbalizes a *picture summary*.

5. The student verbalizes a *word summary*.

6. The student verbalizes the *main idea* from the imaged gestalt.

    a. Stimulate main idea generalizing with the principle of contrast and choice.
    b. Stimulate main idea generalizing by initiating a part of it.

7. The teacher asks "why" questions to stimulate an *inference* from the imaged gestalt.

8. The teacher asks questions from the imaged gestalt that will stimulate the student's ability to *draw conclusions and predict/extend* information.

9. Consider the issue of *lesson energy*.

10. Remember to diagnose for automatic imaging *as* language is received.

11. Remember to require the student to receive language in all three modes: receptive—aloud—to self.

12. **Group Instruction:**
    Consider the small group—3 to 5 students—a collective individual. All students participate in the same paragraph. Choose a different student to 1) visualize and verbalize each sentence, 2) check through structure words on

first sentence, 3) verbalize picture summary and word summary, and 4) respond to interpretive questions.

Chapter 9

Multiple Sentence Imaging

Multiple sentence imaging with higher order thinking skills uses a modified format of the sentence by sentence level and is therefore easily mastered by both teacher and student(s). In sentence by sentence, one sentence was the "part." Now the part will be extended to two sentences, a third, or half the paragraph. The purpose of this step is to continue developing "gestalting" from larger units of language.

The sessions include a picture summary, a word summary, and interpretive comprehension skills. The use of colored squares is recommended.

The lessons are beginning to slim down. Structure words are obsolete. Detailed images are requested only in the initial stages of the multiple sentence level. Students are imaging with a fair amount of automaticity and detail, and the lessons require less questioning from you. The individual is visualizing and verbalizing more easily.

Sometimes lower level material is used in the initial stages of multiple sentence imaging. However, the student may have advanced to higher level material in sentence by sentence and usually continuess at that level now. The content of the material is not yet significant since the goal is to continue developing spontaneous and automatic imaging, not to teach content.

The following sample lesson will demonstrate the reduced amount of questioning required of you. This lesson is with Steve, a 22-year-old college student. His reading comprehension is moderately weak but severely handicapping him in college. He must read material more than once to understand it. He is very verbal and socially successful. Due to his winning personality, it is often difficult to believe that he has problems with language comprehension.

sample lesson 12: Two Sentences x Two Sentences

The paragraph is again from Richard Boning's *Specific Skills*. The text is:

131

> **The mystery of how salmon can find their way back to their home rivers is solved. The salmon navigate by sun and stars when traveling in the ocean. When the salmon nears the general area of the river in which it was born, it uses its nose. The salmon can remember the smell of the home river that it left as a baby.**

Nanci: "This time you will read two sentences aloud, visualize and verbalize, and give a picture summary. You may use a colored square for each sentence."

Steve: "You want me to read it aloud?"

Nanci: "Yes, and try to visualize *AS* you read...then give me a picture summary."

Steve: **"The mystery of how salmon can find their way back to their home rivers is solved. The salmon navigate by sun and stars when traveling in the ocean."**

Nanci: "What do those words make you picture?"

Steve: He places a colored square. "I see salmon swimming in a river. They're on the surface of the water, about three or four of them. I can see their mouths coming out of the water occasionally. It is night, but it is moonlight with lots of stars. When their mouths come up, they sort of look at the stars."

Nanci: "I agree that the first sentence made me see the salmon in the river. Does the second sentence keep the salmon in the river?"

Steve: "Hmmm...let me see...**The salmon navigate by sun and stars when traveling in the ocean.** Oops! Now I can see the salmon in the ocean, their mouths still coming out and they're looking at the stars. It is the same picture only I can see them in the ocean."

Nanci: Concerned that he may not have a strong image for ocean, but may have just paraphrased... "Describe what you see for the ocean. Are the salmon close to shore or way out in the middle of the ocean? Is the water rough or...?"

Steve: "They are getting near some land. They are still pretty far away but you can see some land in the moonlight. The ocean is calm. It seems like a balmy night. Lots of stars, not much wind and the salmon are heading in a certain direction."

Nanci: "Good images. Keep reading and let's see if they get where they're going."

Steve: **"When the salmon nears the general area of the river in which it was born, it uses its nose. The salmon can remember the smell of the home river that it left as a baby.** (He places the second square.) "I see a salmon getting closer to the shore and there is a river emptying into the ocean. Now the salmon has his mouth out of the water, but I can see like a nose near his mouth, with little holes. He sniffs as he swims and goes up the river."

Nanci: "Great images. I see his nose too. Is it still dark but moonlight?"

Steve: "Yes...it is the same ocean and same balmy night, only the salmon became one salmon heading up a river. There are some cliffs around where the river meets the ocean. I can see the outline of them in the moonlight."

Nanci: "Great. Can you see the salmon going further up the river? The sentence said something about a home river that it left as a baby?"

Steve: "Oh yeah. I can see him going up a river with his nose out. There are rocks on the bottom of the river bed and the river is shallow at times so the salmon's nose is sticking up a lot. The river banks are grassy looking, even in the dark, and I see him sort of stopping in front of a large rock and sort of floating there. I can even see him thinking of a little mother salmon waiting for him there."

Nanci: "So can I. She has a little apron on and glasses. (We chuckle...how silly.) Now give me a picture summary."

Steve: Touching the first square... "I saw some salmon swimming in an ocean at night. Lots of stars out, moonlight too, and their mouths kept coming out of the water...then they looked at the stars. They were sort of close to land and were heading in a certain direction. (Touching second square...) Then I saw one of the salmon and he got real close to the land and there was a river emptying into the ocean and he began to twitch his nose and go up the river. He heads up the river, skimming over rocks (gesturing) with his nose out and then he finds a certain big rock and just floats there near it. There is even a little sign that says HOME by the rock."

Nanci: "Great. You even added a few things. Now can you give me a word summary? Just tell the story back to me as if you were the author, but use your images to help you."

Steve: "This story was about how salmon find their way home...."

Nanci: "Wait. Let's start the word summary without saying 'This story was about.' Let's start with 'Salmon find their way....'"

Steve: "Oh...OK. Salmon find their way back to their home river by using the stars to help them navigate when they are in the ocean. That helps them find the general place where the river is that they came from...and when they get close, they smell—use their noses—to help them locate the river where they were born."

Interpretive questions:

Nanci: *Main Idea:* "Good summary! Can you tell me the main idea of this paragraph?"

Steve: "Sure. The main idea is how salmon find their way back to the river where they were born."

Nanci: *Inference:* "I agree. Why did the author initially use the word MYSTERY? He said, 'The mystery is solved.' Why was it a mystery?"

Steve: "It was a mystery because fish can't read maps and yet salmon apparently return to the same river where they were born."

Nanci: *Inference:* "Right. How do you think we even knew that salmon found their way back?"

Steve: "Well, fish and game rangers probably...hmmm...let me see...they must have tagged the salmon when they were born, or marked them in some way and then they could tell if a salmon came back to the same spot."

Nanci: *Conclusion:* "What can we conclude about how salmon feel about their home river?"

I continue to ask a few more questions that require predicting and extending. However, the paragraph is short and a relatively low grade level, so there is not a lot of content from which to work.

Analysis of sample lesson 12

Steve was great, wasn't he? Did you notice how he appeared to be imaging spontaneously and I did not have to provide as many questions. He generated images from the material and was able to describe his images and give a word summary with ease. The multiple sentence level is similar to the sentence by sentence level but the student is visualizing more easily, is able to give good picture and word summaries, and is very comfortable with the concept of main idea. You will not need to ask for quite so much detail and can *begin to assume imaging*.

The use of colored squares is recommended at the multiple sentence level. They do help to anchor the imaged parts and have value as long as the student is giving a picture summary. The picture summaries ascertain that he is actually imaging and give him something concrete from which to verbalize.

It is now very important to be diagnosing if the student is visualizing *as* he receives or reads language. The images should be occurring automatically. Ask yourself a few diagnostic questions. Is the student pausing at the end of the sentences? If so, this means he is not automatically imaging while reading. Is the student returning to a familiar habit of reading very fast, without connecting, and then having to reread to image? This is common, but undesirable, and an indication of further stimulation needed. On the other hand, is the student demonstrating imaging with chuckles, sighs, alarm, or disgust, while reading or listening? If yes, he is probably imaging with some automaticity.

The lesson proceeds in the same manner, despite how the student receives the information. Again, the material should be presented in each mode:

- You read to the student (receptive).
- Student reads aloud (expressive).
- Student reads to self.

If the student is reading silently, try to be certain that he doesn't read it more than once before verbalizing. You are diagnosing if he is imaging while reading the first time through, not the second and third time.

The material should become increasingly more difficult, reaching his oral vocabulary potential and/or grade level.

Practice Multiple Sentence Imaging

Practice and overlap to the next level!

Summary of Multiple Sentence Imaging

step 7

Objective: The student will be able to visualize and verbalize, *with automaticity*, from two or more sentences at a time, verbalizing word summaries and answering higher order thinking skill questions.

1. This step is a modified format of sentence by sentence imaging.

2. The goal is to continue constructing imaged gestalts from larger and larger "parts."

3. The student receives or reads two sentences, a third, or half the paragraph.

4. *The structure words are obsolete.*

5. The use of the colored squares is recommended.

6. Include a picture summary.

7. Include a word summary to generalize the imaged gestalt.

8. The student will visualize and verbalize more easily now and require less questioning and stimulation.

9. Note whether the student is visualizing and verbalizing with automaticity *as* the language enters his or her mind.

10. Ask interpretive comprehension questions of *main idea, inference, conclusion, prediction.*

11. Use all three modes of receiving language: receptive, aloud, self.

12. **Group Instruction:**
    Choose a different student to 1) V/V each part of the paragraph, 2) give the picture summary, 3) give the word summary, and 4) answer interpretive questions.

Chapter 10

Whole Paragraph Imaging

Take a deep breath. The "part" has increased to a whole paragraph. Now the student receives or reads an entire paragraph without pausing, all the while visualizing and verbalizing. There is no need for colored squares nor a formal picture summary. The student will give a word summary only, but you question for specific images, just to be confident that imaging is continuing. *You must ask interpretive comprehension questions.*

The V/V process takes less time now since there is less need for questioning and stimulation. However, *begin to refine the student's verbalization.* Request that the student be explicit in word summaries. Call attention to redundant phrases and use of pronouns that cause image confusion.

Each paragraph requires less time to complete, so include at least three to five paragraphs in each lesson. I continue using the Boning *Specific Skills* books, which have self-contained, high-imagery paragraphs.

It is important to continue diagnosing for spontaneous, automatic imagery *as* the information is entering the mind. Use all three modes of receiving language: receptive, read aloud, read to self. Note gesturing, eye movements, laughter or any responses that indicate images are being constructed from the language.

---

sample lesson 13: Whole Paragraph

The following sample lesson will be with Jerry, our sixth-grade boy, who has now progressed to the whole paragraph level. Recall that although his decoding of words ranged from a ninth-to a 12th-grade level, his comprehension was unstable at the third-grade level. In this lesson he will read a whole paragraph aloud from a sixth-grade skill book and comprehend it. He still tries to wear his army fatigue cap in every session. The paragraph is again from Richard Boning's *Specific Skills*. The text is:

> **There is a worm in the sea that is actually a living fishline! This is the fishline worm. It can be found curled up under a rock. It looks small, but when it uncoils it is eighty feet long. The sharp teeth of the worm attach themselves to a small fish. Once they do, they never let go. Finally the fish tires of fighting the long worm. The fishline worm then devours its catch.**

Nanci: "Jerry, this time I want you to read the whole paragraph aloud to me. Remember to image as you read and when you are through give me a word summary."

Jerry: **"There is a worm in the sea that is actually a living fishline! This is the fishline worm. It can be found curled up under a rock. It looks small, but when it uncoils it is eighty feet long. The sharp teeth of the worm attach themselves to a small fish. Once they do, they never let go. Finally the fish tires of fighting the long worm. The fishline worm then devours its catch."**

Nanci: "Did you get some images for that? I did!"

Jerry: "Yes. I saw a long worm on the bottom of the ocean. It is curled up near a rock. The ocean is kind of greenish-blue and there are fish swimming around. This worm springs out at a fish and eats it."

Nanci: "Good imaging. Read from here (pointing to the paragraph) and see if you want to add anything to or change your images in any way."

Jerry: **"It looks small, but when it uncoils it is eighty feet long. The sharp teeth of the worm attach themselves to a small fish.** (Pause) **Once they do, they never let go. Finally the fish tires of fighting the long worm. The fishline worm then devours its catch....** Oh, now I see the worm's mouth and some pointed sharp teeth. When he springs at the fish, he grabs on with his teeth. The fish keeps pulling away, like this (gesturing), but the worm hangs on. The fish gets real tired and the worm eats it with its sharp teeth."

Nanci: "That's what I saw, too. Only I see something about the worm that is unusual. For instance, what does the worm look like, besides having pointed, sharp teeth?"

Jerry: "It is like a worm...it is shaped like a worm and is long."

Nanci: "How long is it?"

Jerry: "80 feet."

Nanci: "Right. Can you imagine how long 80 feet would be?"

Jerry: "Hmm...about from this side of the room to that side?"

Nanci: "That would be about 15 feet. Eighty feet would be from here to across the street to that tree."

Jerry: "Oh! That worm was that long?... And, he just stays all coiled up and then wears out the fish...like on a fishing line."

Nanci: "Now I think you really have a good image of that paragraph. Give me a word summary and begin with 'There is an unusual worm called the....' "

Jerry: "There is an unusual worm called the fishline worm. He is just like a real fishing line. He is real long and lives in the ocean. He stays under a rock, all coiled up and when a fish goes by he grabs on to it with his sharp teeth. He hangs on to the fish with his teeth until the fish gets tired. Then he eats it."

Higher order thinking questions

Main Idea:

Nanci: "Excellent. What was the main idea?"

Jerry: "The main idea was that there is a worm called the fishline worm that catches fish just like a fishing line does."

Inference:

Nanci: "Right. Why did they call it a fishline worm?"

Jerry: "Because...it is real long, like a fishing line and it has teeth like a fish hook so it catches fish just like a fishline."

Nanci: "If the worm didn't eat the fish right away—could the worm ever be in danger?"

Jerry: "Hmm...well, I can see it all stretched out on the bottom of the ocean floor and the fish is struggling on the other end and maybe it would be cut in half, or something."

Nanci: "What is the 'it' that might get cut in half? The fish or the worm? I'm not sure what to image."

Jerry: "I meant the worm might get cut in part by another fish that came along and ate the worm...or by catching itself on a sharp rock as the fish pulled at one end."

Nanci: "Right. I was also picturing that another fish might come along and try to eat the fishline worm! In fact, there is something unusual about this story in terms of who eats who. Can you tell me what is unusual?"

Jerry: "Well, I usually think of a fish eating a worm, not a worm eating a fish!"

We chuckled and pursued some other interpretive comprehension questions such as:

1. *Inference:*
   Based on the story, how thick do you think the worm would have to be? Why?

2. *Predict/extend:*
   How often do you think the worm might need to catch a fish? Why?

3. *Inference:*
   What size fish do you think the worm catches? Why?

4. *Draw conclusion:*
   What can we conclude about the teeth of this worm? Why?

5. *Predict/extend:*
   Based on all these images, what do you think would happen if you were fishing near a fishline worm?

Note: All the above questions use the imaged gestalt as the base from which to process.

The whole paragraph level omits structure words, colored squares, and a picture summary. A word summary is usually the first description the student gives after reading or hearing a paragraph. Continue some questioning to be assured of imaging. He may describe his images in entirety, or you may want to have him describe a significant aspect of the content.

If material is omitted in the verbalization, it usually means that it has not been imaged. When this happens, simply have the student reread part or all the selection. Don't provide the images. After rereading a section, it is common to hear him say, "Oh, I didn't picture that part."

Preface the rereading activity with a challenge to the student to see if he needs to *add* or *change* the image in any way. For example, Jerry had not imaged the middle section of the paragraph well and I requested that he reread to check if he needed to add or change images. It is completely appropriate, and important, for the student to reread to create or improve images. Many students have acquired a habit of tuning out language by either not focusing or reading too rapidly. They need to break that "tuning-out" habit by replacing it with a "tuning-in" habit. It is likely that the process of connecting to language was so slow and laborious that they acquired an unconscious habit that is often difficult to break. It is an encouraging sign for the student to spontaneously reread in order to image. It means "tuning-out" is beginning to wane.

At the whole paragraph level, you *check* to determine if the individual is imaging. The questioning is less than at the sentence by sentence level, but often appropriate. In the previous lesson, Jerry didn't image the length of the worm because he didn't have a good concept of distance. This is not unusual; the concept of distance is frequently a weakness for students with poor imagery. Five inches can be interpreted as half an inch...or six feet. I needed to question and be sure Jerry imaged the concept of distance that was quite important to the story.

It is vital to continue to develop inferring, predicting, concluding, and evaluating skills from whole paragraph processing. The reason for this stimulation was to develop higher order thinking skills from oral and written language. Don't omit it now.

Practice Whole Paragraph Imaging

Practice, practice, practice, and then overlap. Increase the level of material as is appropriate.

Paragraph Imaging

1. Jerry visualizes while reading a paragraph.

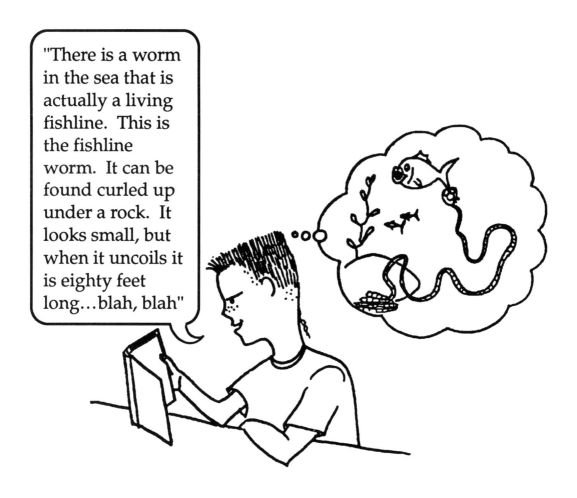

"There is a worm in the sea that is actually a living fishline. This is the fishline worm. It can be found curled up under a rock. It looks small, but when it uncoils it is eighty feet long…blah, blah"

2. Nanci questions and Jerry gives a "word summary."

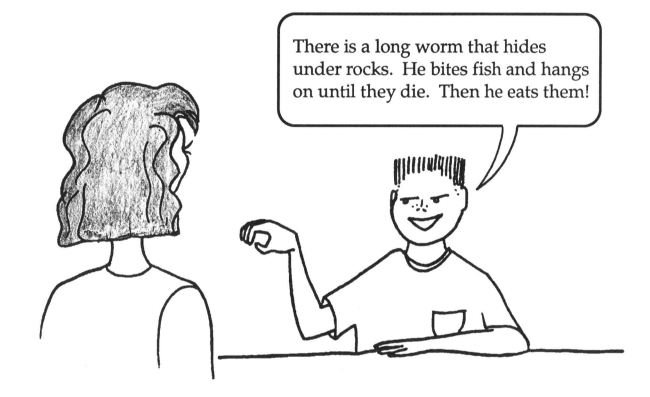

Summary of Whole Paragraph Imaging

step 8

Objective: The student will be able to visualize and verbalize a whole paragraph with automaticity, refined verbal summaries, and good interpretive higher order comprehension.

1. This step modifies the format of previous levels, thus is easily mastered by all.

2. The student reads and/or receives a whole paragraph of content.

3. *No colored squares or structure words are necessary.*

4. *No picture summary.* Instead, the student describes specific images *after* giving a word summary.

5. The student verbalizes a *refined* word summary.

6. **Ask interpretive comprehension questions to be answered from the imaged gestalt.**

   - **Main idea**
   - **Inference**
   - **Conclusion**
   - **Predict/extend**
   - **Evaluate**

7. Diagnose whether the student is imaging automatically. Note gesturing, eye movement, or response to content as the individual receives language.

8. Use all three modes of receiving language:

   - receptive—you read to the student
   - expressive—student reads aloud
   - expressive— student reads to self

9. The student may reread all or part of the content in order to image.

10. Although imaging is more automatic and assumed at this level, question specifics to determine that the individual is actually imaging and not just restating sentences or paraphrasing.

11. **Group Instruction:**
One student reads or receives the entire paragraph and gives a word summary. Teacher and other students question for imaging. Students take turns responding to interpretive questions.

Chapter 11

Paragraph by Paragraph Imaging

Now able to process an entire paragraph of content, the student is ready to begin *paragraph by paragraph imaging*. This step is very similar to sentence by sentence imaging in that the individual will read or receive a number of parts to create the gestalt. In sentence by sentence, the parts were the sentences and the gestalt was the paragraph. In paragraph by paragraph imaging, the parts are the paragraphs and the gestalt is the page.

The procedure is simple. Have the student read or receive an entire paragraph and give a word summary for that paragraph. You may want to check imaging by just asking the student what was pictured for certain parts, but now you are assuming imaging and refining verbal summaries. Continue with each paragraph on the page and then have the student give a generalized succinct summary of the entire page—a *page summary*.

The use of colored squares is optional. Squares may be placed for text with six or fewer paragraphs. The student can touch each square for the generalized page summary to help retrieve the images and the general content of each paragraph. Do not request a picture summary for each one.

The following sample lesson is with Cindy, a fourth-grade girl who was almost retained in third grade. Instead, she received auditory conceptual tutoring and Visualizing/Verbalizing in the summer, and by November was handling fourth-grade work. She is brunette, skinny, and very active.

_____

sample lesson 14: Paragraph by Paragraph Imaging

Nanci: **"Now we will begin to visualize and verbalize a whole page of material** (the student gasps), **but we will do it paragraph by paragraph so that it won't be difficult. You can read the first paragraph aloud, place a colored square, and then give me a word summary of the paragraph. When you are all through with each paragraph, you can tell me about the whole page you read!"**

Cindy read the entire text from Richard Boning's *Specific Skills*. The text is:

The Elephant Bird

The first people who visited Africa came back with strange stories. Their stories were about a giant bird. The name of the bird was the elephant bird.

The elephant bird was very large. One story told how it could eat baby elephants. Another story told how the bird would drop rocks on ships that passed by. Still another story told of how the bird carried a person away in its claws! People liked to hear such stories, but not all of them were true. People began to wonder. Was the elephant bird real? "No bird could grow that large," people said.

Today we know for a fact that the elephant bird really did live. How do we know? Bones of the bird have been found. The bones were dug out of the ground on an island near Africa. Eggshells of the elephant bird have also been found.

The bones show that the elephant bird was a giant, taller than the tallest human being. It was ten feet high. It was also very heavy. An elephant bird often weighed a thousand pounds. The eggs of the elephant bird were the largest eggs ever laid—the size of basketballs. People who find the eggshells today make them into water jugs. The jugs can hold over eight quarts of water.

No one knows how the elephant bird got it's name. We do know that it was too heavy to fly, so not all the stories about it are true. Did it really eat baby elephants? We do not know, but why do you think it was called the elephant bird?

Analysis of paragraph 1:

Cindy read the first paragraph aloud. She placed a colored square and gave a word summary. I checked to be sure she was imaging by checking for specific, important images. For example, "What did you see for the giant bird?"

Analysis of paragraph 2:

Cindy read the second paragraph. She had more images, placed a colored square for the paragraph, and began verbalizing a word summary and gesturing her images. She imaged a bird that was almost as big as her and she saw it trying to eat a baby elephant. She quickly added, though, that she didn't think this was a true story. Then, gesturing, she described her image of this big bird flying over a ship in the ocean and dropping a great big boulder on the ship. Continuing, she proceeded to describe that the same bird picked up a person in his huge claws (gesturing) and carried the person away (more gesturing).

Analysis of paragraph 3:

She read the third paragraph, placed another square, and gave a word summary. When I checked, she had fewer images this time. She just imaged people digging and finding large bones and large eggs in the sand. We interacted to stimulate her imagery.

Analysis of paragraph 4:

She read the fourth paragraph, showed lots of reaction as she read, and placed another square. Her word summary was good. This time she included lots of images. She began enthusiastically describing a bird that was bigger than me. We discussed the 10-foot ceilings in my office and the bird being that tall. She imagined a huge bird! Then she described a big egg. She wasn't sure of the size of a basketball, so I showed her a make-believe one with my hands. By this time, she was completely absorbed in the paragraph and couldn't wait to read more.

Analysis of paragraph 5:

She started to read the last paragraph, but I stopped her after the first sentence and asked her how she thought the elephant bird got its name. Obviously imaging, we hypothesized that the bird was really large like an elephant. I asked her why they didn't call it a "hippo bird" or some other jungle animal that was large. Thinking and imaging again, she thought that perhaps the bird was a gray color and had a really long beak like an elephant's trunk.

We continued. She read this sentence: **We do know that it was too heavy to fly, so not all the stories about it are true.** I stopped her again and asked her which stories she thought weren't true. She moved her eyes up, indicating imaging, and then said, "Oh, the bird couldn't fly so he didn't throw rocks at the ship and he didn't really carry people away." Note that she retrieved her sensory information—images— from the first paragraph in order to answer the interpretive comprehension question.

She finished reading the rest of the paragraph and placed a square. She then verbalized that the bird was so heavy that she saw it trying and trying to fly by flapping his huge wings, but he was never able to get off the ground. We discussed whether we really thought the bird could eat baby elephants. We decided that if it was 10 feet high perhaps it could eat baby elephants...we didn't like to picture that! She decided that was why it was named the "elephant bird" and not the "hippo bird."

Beginning a page summary

She had visualized and verbalized each paragraph and placed colored squares. Now she went back, touched each square to recall her images, and gave me a succinct, interesting, and comprehensive *page summary.* I asked her inference, prediction, and conclusion questions. She consistently returned to her images to help her answer the questions and expanded on the answers without encouragement. "And this could happen...and this could have been the reason...and if this happened, then...." She was responding to print in the same manner that I had seen *good comprehenders* respond. She was reacting, interacting, and generating as she read. One would not have known that she had previously experienced difficulty with reading comprehension.

She was processing language—through images—*as* she read. Images were her sensory connection to language. The continuing sessions reinforced her automaticity of imaging. She read from different levels and different types of material, ranging from high imagery to her content areas in school. She actually had a different light about her face.

The above lesson also used the Boning *Specific Skills* material for a whole page of processing. This material ranges from first- to twelfth- grade level and has high imagery stories. Other material that is useful for a whole page of content is Walter Pauk's *Six Way Paragraphs*. This material ranges from eighth to twelfth grade and the page of material is shorter than in the Boning *Specific Skills*. One of the advantages of Pauk's material is that it incorporates good written comprehension questions that the student can read and answer. However, these written questions are only supplemental to the oral questions continuing to be asked.

The following is a sample page from Pauk. Note the imagery still present even in twelfth-grade material.

Beyond the Call of Duty

The marathon, a regular event in the Olympic Games, got its name from the Greek plain of Marathon, where a battle between the Persian army led by King Darius, and the Athenian army was fought in 490 B.C.

Darius's troops had arrived on Marathon and were preparing to attack Athens. The Athenians were greatly outnumbered by the Persians, so they sent a runner, Pheidippides, to Sparta to request aid against the attackers. Pheidippides ran 140 miles to Sparta in about twenty-four hours. After receiving a promise of help from the Spartans, he ran back to deliver the news, again covering the rocky terrain in twenty-four hours.

Pheidippides fought in the battle of Marathon several days later. The Spartans didn't come to their aid in time, but the Athenians were victorious anyway. The commander of the army wanted to notify the citizens of Athens of the Persians' defeat. The battle-weary Pheidippides, who had had little time to recover from his 280-mile run of the previous week, agreed to be the messenger.

He set off on the nearly twenty-five-mile-long trek from Marathon to Athens, and ran into the Athenian marketplace just a few hours later. He gasped "Rejoice, we conquer," then dropped dead in his tracks before the astounded onlookers.

The marathon footrace was established as an Olympic event in honor of Pheidippides. The official distance for a marathon is 26 miles, 385 yards.

The student reads each paragraph, images, might place a colored square, and verbalizes a word summary for each paragraph, just as in the previous lesson with Cindy. Then, after completing the entire page, the student gives a page summary, answers oral questions, and then answers Pauk's written questions.

Analysis of paragraph by paragraph imaging

Paragraph by paragraph imaging is quite simple. There are a few but critical changes.

Use colored squares when you have fewer than six paragraphs. If you don't use the squares, the page summary will probably be less precise, less sequential, and less specific. Therefore, in the initial stages of paragraph by paragraph, it would be best to use material that lends itself to the use of colored squares. This will help control the sequence and flow of the page summary and actually develop the processing—gestalting—of more information.

At this level, the student is receiving language orally or by reading either aloud or silently. It is important to increase silent reading since most comprehension of written material will be from silent reading, not oral reading! Continue to include receptive input—reading to the student—in order to continue facilitating oral language processing.

Vocabulary becomes an important issue in determining the grade level of the paragraphs to image. Use the student's oral vocabulary as a base measure of potential, but remember that vocabulary can be developed by imaging content. For example, the student can derive the meaning of a word based on the surrounding *imaged* context. In the later stages of V/V, I often move into material that challenges the student's vocabulary. This illustrates the direct relationship between imaging and vocabulary, and helps the student begin to recognize the need for using a dictionary, or questioning the teacher/parent for the definition of a given word—all in order to image content. When she begins to stop and ask the meaning of certain words, I am confident that she is reading for meaning and not just reading words.

Practice Paragraph by Paragraph Imaging

The goal at the paragraph by paragraph level is automatic imaging; a succinct, specific page summary; and accurate responses to interpretive, higher order comprehension questions of main idea, inference, conclusion, prediction, and evaluation. Practice until the above is achieved and then overlap to more difficult and dense material, and the next level of processing.

Paragraph by Paragraph Imaging

1. Cindy reads each paragraph and visualizes/verbalizes.

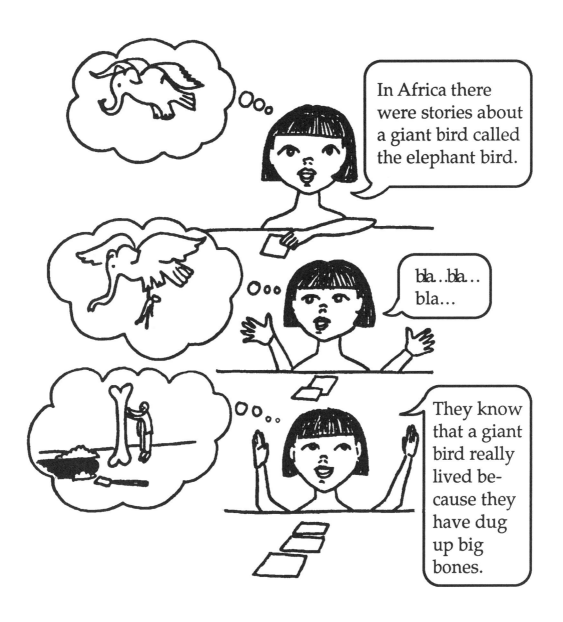

2. Cindy gives a word summary for each paragraph.

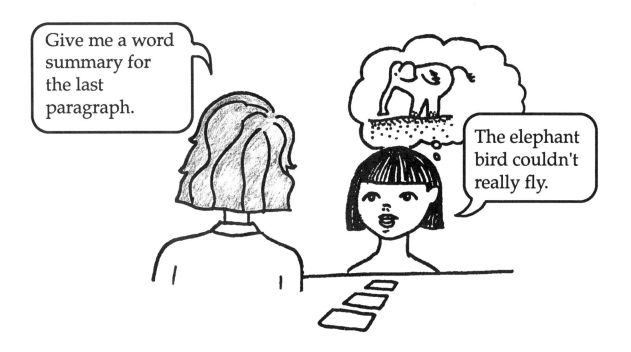

3. Using her imaged gestalt, Cindy answers interpretive comprehension questions.

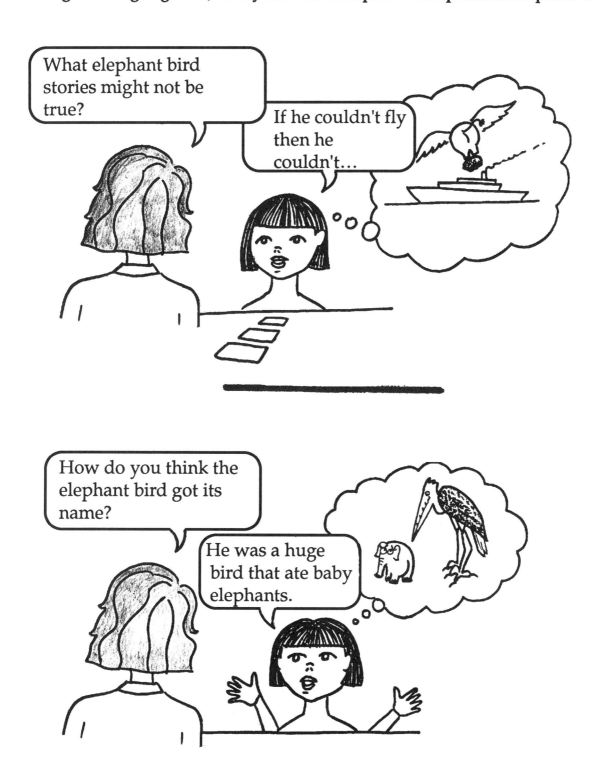

Summary of Paragraph by Paragraph Imaging

step 9

Objective: The student will be able to visualize and verbalize a whole page of written material (one paragraph at a time), give a general page summary, and answer interpretive, higher order comprehension questions.

1. The student receives or reads entire paragraph.

2. The student verbalizes a word summary per paragraph, placing a colored square.

3. The teacher checks for specific images, but primarily assumes imaging.

4. The student touches each colored square and gives a *page summary* of the entire page of material.

5. The student reads aloud or silently, with the emphasis on the latter. Include receptive stimulation to continue aiding the student in processing oral language.

6. *It is imperative to continue interpretive questions of main idea, inference, conclusion, prediction, and evaluation.*

7. **Group Instruction:**
   Each student reads or receives one paragraph, places a colored square, and gives paragraph word summary. Choose one student to give a page summary and different students to answer interpretive questions.

Chapter 12

Whole Page Imaging

The Visualizing/Verbalizing process has finally arrived at a *whole page* of comprehension work. Isn't it remarkable to think that most instruction in reading comprehension begins here and assumes comprehension of whole paragraphs or whole pages when just isolated words are taught? In fact, most instruction assumes comprehension of whole chapters. Hence, the plight of Catherine. We often expect not only pages but chapters of information to be processed, stored, recalled, retrieved, applied, and tested without direct instruction in reading comprehension.

The whole page imaging level is the final step preparatory to chapter processing. The teaching techniques of whole page imaging vary only slightly from the previous level. The sentence by sentence level stimulated and established the student's ability to image parts to whole. This developed the gestalt base from which all other comprehension and thinking skills are processed. Although the technique at the whole page level is not different, it is critical to include this step in order to apply imaging to content, and larger and larger "parts" of information.

Learn from my mistakes. In the early stages of developing this V/V process, I discontinued the work past the whole paragraph level. I assumed that students would automatically apply their imaging and comprehension skills to a whole page of material and to whole chapters of content. I learned, however, that they might return to the same ingrained habit of reading very fast, "tuning-out," and not imaging/connecting to the language. This whole page level prevents that and *is not to be omitted.*

Whole page imaging is an entire page of visualizing and verbalizing. The colored squares are not used. Detailed imagery is not requested for each sentence or paragraph. You may request some images throughout the page, but be aware that detailed imagery will make the sessions too lengthy. Assume imagery and note if the student is interacting with the language, moving eyes upward, or defocusing.

In the following lesson, Jerry will simply read or receive an entire page and give a page summary and respond to questions that stimulate his ability to reason.

sample lesson 15: Whole Page Imaging

The following lesson is from Boning's *Specific Skills*, "Getting the Facts."

The Tree-Climbing Fish
What would you think if you saw a fish walking along? Would you take another look if you saw a fish climbing a tree? There is a fish that does both of these things. It is called the Tree-Climbing Fish.

A traveler to India first told about the Tree-Climbing Fish. The fish was high up in a tree. What was the fish doing in the tree? How did it get there? The traveler thought a bird might have put it there.

The next day the traveler saw a fish come out of the water. It was hard to believe, but up the road it went. The fish used its fins and tail to push itself along. It stopped to eat some worms. After the fish had eaten, it walked over to a tree. Up, up it climbed. When it got high up in the tree, it took a rest.

The traveler was surprised to see these things and told other people about the Tree-Climbing Fish. The people wanted to know how this fish looked. "The Tree-Climbing Fish is not too big," said the traveler. "It is often about ten inches long. It is dark brown in color."

Children of India like to catch this fish. They can go fishing in their own backyards. They just wait for the fish to come walking by!

Jerry read the entire page to himself and gave me a page summary. He summarized the page, using images to support his organization and verbalization. I checked for imaging and *asked interpretive comprehension questions*. We then completed the lesson by answering the written questions that accompany that page of content.

It is that simple. If he experiences difficulty or demonstrates weak images, I include sentence by sentence and multiple sentence imaging in each of his sessions—while continuing whole page imaging. I simply overlap backward.

The student should read silently at the whole page imaging level if accurate decoding is not an issue. If working with high school or college students, I also use the GED and SAT practice manuals for material that is more complex and dense. The passages of reading comprehension practice are usually two to five paragraphs and have good written interpretive comprehension questions.

It is noticeable now that the sessions have slimmed down in terms of questioning to stimulate imagery. An imaged gestalt is assumed and practiced with larger and larger units of language. The student is now automatically interpreting the content, preferably without prompting or questioning from you. *The primary goal is to refine verbalization and critical thinking skills.*

Practice Whole Page Imaging

The term *practice and overlap* still applies here. Look for *refined verbalization* and good response to interpretive questions. Overlap to denser material, especially content areas from school work. Overlap backward if you note weak images.

Summary of Whole Page Imaging

step 10

Objective: The student will be able to visualize and verbalize a page of written material, give a *refined* page summary, and answer oral and written interpretive comprehension questions.

1. V/V continues with larger and larger units of language—a whole page.

2. Detailed imagery is not necessary unless there is some question as to whether the student is not imaging automatically.

3. The student verbalizes a *refined* page summary.

4. The student is moved into higher grade levels as well as denser and different types of material. Extend to content areas.

5. The primary focus is on silent reading, but pursue some receptive stimulation to continue stimulating oral language comprehension and prepare for note taking lectures.

6. The student is now *automatically* interpreting the content, preferably without prompting or questioning. ***The goal is to refine verbalization and higher order thinking skills.***

Chapter 13

Noting: Chapter & Lecture

The individual, dependent upon age and need, now extends his or her skills to application to content through *chapter and lecture noting*. Noting develops comprehension for lengthy, abstract material and/or chapters of content. The student will learn to take notes. If you are not working with students in school, then you may want to omit note-taking but still have individuals read longer and denser material to extend and apply their newly learned comprehension skills to abstract and/or numerous pages of information. A magazine article or a chapter in a book will suffice.

If you are working with students attending school, chapter and lecture noting should be developed. Again, learn from my experience because this is also a step that I previously didn't include with every student. I assumed that the student would automatically apply newly learned comprehension skills to chapter study or that chapter study was included in school instruction. Neither case is always true. Many students don't automatically apply their new comprehension skills thoroughly nor are study skills a part of every class.

Working remedially with high school and college students in the V/V process made it obvious that they rarely had good study techniques. For example, when they were comfortable with the whole page level and I checked their application to school work, they would regress to the old habit of preparing for a test by just reading and rereading chapters. Sitting across from Steve who only months before had been unable to comprehend a short paragraph, I realized that it would be impossible for him to just read and then expect to remember whole chapters of content for an exam. Even with good comprehension, that would be difficult!

The best method for storing, learning, and retrieving large blocks of content is to take notes. **Chapter notes generalize and summarize written material to a reduced state that can be learned, memorized, stored, interpreted, and retrieved.**

Although a simple process, chapter noting can be very difficult for students. Begin by explaining to the student that the purpose of taking chapter notes is to read a chapter once and be prepared for an exam. Further explain that by noting the chapter, 10 to 15 pages of material can be reduced to only a few pages of notes...and these notes can be learned and memorized. All this equals good grades on exams.

First have the student scan the chapter to get an overall image of the information. To scan means to read titles and headings, and perhaps the first sentence in each paragraph. In other words, peruse the chapter for *preparatory images*. Then read and take notes.

Unfortunately, it is often not that simple. The student will either write down everything or will write down nothing! She will either transcribe the entire chapter or write down only the headings. Chapter noting can be particularly difficult for students who have only recently learned to comprehend a body of material. Therefore, teach *what* to include by using V/V to determine the main idea and relevant details. Then teach *how* to include it by modeling the noting process.

Do not teach formal outlining. Instead, teach a noting technique of a general, modified outline of *indenting, enlarging, listing,* and *using the equal sign and the colon,* as described below:

1. Construct a very **general outline** of the information. Sometimes it is appropriate to outline with headings of roman numerals, capital letters, and numbers—a lose version of a formal outline. Or, sometimes it is appropriate to make a very informal outline by just enlarging the main idea and following it with indented details.

2. **Indent details** under the main idea.

3. **Enlarge** dates, names, definitions, or key concepts.

4. **List** information to be memorized.

5. **Use an equal sign** for definitions **or a colon** for concepts related to a specific thought.

The following is an actual example of the chapter notes from a high school senior before I taught her my noting technique. Although she knew *what* to include (she had the basic ideas), she didn't know *how* to include it. **Note how difficult it would be to study this information.**

Chapter 36

Work for youth-two agencies were created to bring immediate relief to youth, 1933 the Civilian Conservation Corps (CCS) 500,000 young men between 18 & 25 enrolled in the CCC, the young Americans did socially useful work. The second agency was the National Youth Administration (NYA) created in 1935 distributed federal money to needy students in its 1st yr the NYA gave 400,00 jobs to students, these 2 agencies helped hundreds of thousands of students get an education maintain their self-respect.

Blacks and the New Deal-Blacks were still discriminated against after the war. They had the hardest time with the relief agencies, they had the lowest working rates.

She had all the correct ideas but it was not in a format that could be studied. The following is another example of the same material using a modified noting technique. Notice how much easier it will be to store and retrieve this information.

Chap. 36
*   I. Work for youth*
*   2 agencies:*
CCC: *NYA:*
Civilian Conservation Corps   *National Youth Agency*
1. 1933   *1. 1935*
2. 500,000 men (18-25 yrs)   *2. $ to needy students*
3. most unmarried   *3. regular wages*
4. most poverty   *4. 400,000 student*
5. lived in work camps   *5. prevented idleness*
6. given: food, clothing   *6. Kept youth out of*
7. paid wages-Families   *overcrowded job market*
8. opportunities for Ed.
9. did useful work

Practice Chapter Noting

Teach and practice the format of a modified outline with listing, indenting, and enlarging. Usually this step requires quite a lot of practice. Start with the student verbalizing *what* to include while you model *how* to include it by noting in the above technique. Then you tell the student what to include and the student writes

171

the notes. Move to you and the student each noting an area and comparing which notes would be easily studied. Practice until the student can quickly, accurately, and informally outline written information. Overlap to lecture noting.

Lecture Noting

Lecture noting is easily implemented now because you have developed gestalt imagery, language comprehension, higher order thinking skills, and a *noting procedure from written language.*

Begin by exploring with the student the difference between noting written language and noting oral language. Help him recognize the *speed* with which language is expressed and received orally, and that although you can ask for information to be repeated, *there is no opportunity to reread.* Consequently, unique to noting oral language is the importance of quick, accurate analysis of the critical features to note and the need for *brevity* in the note taking process.

Next, give the student experience using the same noting procedure established for chapter noting. Explain that *the same procedure for noting what you read can be applied to noting what you hear.* Begin by reading a whole page of information to him, but modify—deformalize—written language to simulate a lecture. This may mean pausing, adding appropriate verbal analogies, illustrating points on a chalkboard, etc. Instruct him to jot down the highlights. Because of the speed of oral language, he will need to trigger on main ideas, important facts, image examples—and he will need to learn to ask questions.

Questions. The student needs to get comfortable asking for clarity by examples—*imaginal representations.* Not all instructors lecture well and not all illustrate on a chalkboard or overhead transparency. Explore with the student whether he should just let a concept go by or should get his hand up with, "Can you illustrate that point?" Prepare him to ask the instructor to clarify with an example and also prepare him to create his own imaginal representation from an instructor's verbal analogy. For example, in a biology lecture the concept of *symbiosis* is presented. The student needs to learn to generate in his notes an imaginal representation such as "*Symbiosis - 2 organisms support one another in a specific biological environment, i.e., a bee and a flower.*" This is an anchoring process when going from the abstract to the imaginal.

To review the student's notes, you examine and interact regarding the content, explore the strengths and weakness, and note any consistent gaps that will require specific attention in the next practice session. Continue practicing lecture noting with whole pages of information extended to mock lectures of 5 to 10 minutes. Again, the easiest way to simulate a lecture is to deformalize written language from content area chapters.

Chapter and lecture noting stimulation should be offered to students as early as seventh or eighth grade.

Summary

The V/V process taught the comprehension skills that prepared individuals for knowing *what* to include, and now you have to teach them *how* to include it.

- Explain *why* chapter noting is relevant to the student.

- Teach how to *scan* for preparatory images.

- Teach to read and discern *major concepts to be noted*.

- Teach a *noting format* that may be easily learned, stored, and retrieved.

- Follow these simple steps for noting written language:

  1. Student verbalizes what to include, you write the notes.
  2. You verbalize what to include, student writes the notes.
  3. You and student each read and write notes, comparing which would be easier to study.
  4. Student reads and notes, you only give feedback.

- Once the written language noting procedures are fairly well developed, extend to oral language noting.

- Follow these simple steps for noting oral language:

  1. Explore the difference between noting chapters and lectures, resulting in recognition for brief, accurate noting.
  2. Begin practice from one page of material, extending to mock lectures.
  3. Modify written language to simulate a lecture by deformalizing the language and giving examples.
  4. Review the notes, interacting and recognizing areas of further attention.
  5. Explore the need to ask questions for points of clarification or examples.
  6. Remember that imaginal representations serve to anchor abstract material.

Summary of Chapter and Lecture Noting

step 11

Objective: The student will apply V/V to noting oral and written material by analyzing and capturing critical concepts for further study or memorization.

1. Notes reduce content to a size that can be learned, memorized, and retrieved.

2. Explain the need for chapter noting:

   a. Read a chapter only once for an exam.
   b. Reduce numerous pages of content to only a few pages.

3. Scan the chapter for preparatory images.

4. Teach a modified outline technique:

   a. Use general outline of headings or lists.
   b. Indent details.
   c. Enlarge specifics.
   d. List information to be memorized.
   e. Use equal sign or colon.w

5. Model and practice the noting procedure for written language.

   a. Student verbalizes what to include, you write the notes.
   b. You verbalize what to include, student writes the notes.
   c. You and student each read and write notes, comparing which would be easier to study.
   d. Student reads and notes, you give feedback.

6. Extend to practicing noting oral language.

   a. Explore difference between noting oral and written language.
   b. Explore need for brevity in note taking, questioning for example, and need to create imaginal representations.
   c. Deformalize written language for lecturing, begin with one page and extend to mock lectures of 5 to 10 minutes.
   d. Review students' notes, interact, recognize areas of strength and weakness.
   e. Practice, practice, practice....

Chapter 14

Writing from Visualizing and Verbalizing

Y ou must learn to think before you can write. Grammar, punctuation, and spelling aside, you must have organized thoughts in order to write. Without the ability to think—rational, organized, lucid thoughts—writing is unorganized, disjointed, non-specific, and rambling. To teach grammar, punctuation, and spelling, but not teach thinking, is teaching the "parts" but not the "whole."

Visualizing/Verbalizing teaches the "whole" necessary, indeed critical, to writing. If oral and written language comprehension, oral language expression, and thinking are not taught prior to teaching writing, then we must be assuming that some other source is developing these skills. Or, we must be assuming that these skills will be automatically learned from just being alive. Neither may be true so it is necessary to teach them and include them in the school curriculum. Currently, writing instruction in the classroom, from elementary to college, often focuses more on the mechanics of writing than the development of thought process. Perhaps this is because we have not been sure of how to teach thinking, comprehension, and oral language expression. For example, in elementary schools we often focus writing instruction on grammar, spelling, punctuation, and some organization. In high school, we often focus writing instruction on grammar, punctuation, some organization, and not spelling (we assume that spelling was taught in the elementary grades). In college, we often continue instruction on grammar and punctuation, less on spelling, and more focus on organization (although we would like to assume that writing was taught prior to college).

Although we teach writing organization in college, we usually instruct from written language rather than from oral language. For example, we have students note that *their writing* is too general and not specific. We instruct from the written language gestalt rather than from the oral language gestalt.

Many students with language comprehension weakness also have poor writing skill. Attempts to teach them writing are hampered by their comprehension weakness. Here is an example of a college graduate, named Dolores, who conquered her severe reading comprehension and writing disability by using the V/V program as the foundation to develop comprehension/thinking. Her story is not unique.

Dolores was in her early forties, of Mexican descent, a college graduate, employed in a managerial position, and had been trying to pass the California Test of Basic Skills (CBEST) to obtain her teaching credential. She heard me present the Visualizing/Verbalizing theory at a conference on learning disabilities. After my presentation she talked with me concerning her own difficulty with reading comprehension. She explained that she had weakness in reading comprehension and had failed the reading comprehension component of the CBEST test a number of times. If she didn't pass the test, she would be unable to teach. We scheduled her for diagnostic testing.

The testing indicated that Dolores was bright, had adequate oral vocabulary skills, moderate dysfunction in auditory conceptualization, moderate spelling problems, adequate decoding in context, and a severe reading comprehension disability. Although she could read adult level paragraphs with good decoding, she lacked recall of the content. In fact, her comprehension was unstable after the fifth grade paragraph. Did she visualize? No. She got a few "parts" of what she read but no gestalt.

We began V/V treatment. She was an active, interested participant and understood the necessity for developing her visualizing skill. She knew that "words were going in one ear and out the other." As treatment progressed she told me that she also had failed the writing component of the CBEST test. In fact, she failed it with a lower score than the reading comprehension subtest.

I had her write a page or two. Her punctuation, grammar, and spelling were adequate, but the content was non-specific, rambling, and generally very unorganized and difficult to follow. Her writing could be described as lineal. Lineal writing, in exaggerated form, is something like this: "The yellow bus carried children to school...Yellow is a sunny color...Sun is bad for your skin...." This incohesiveness alone would have prevented her from passing the test, but her most debilitating writing weakness was one I should have anticipated, but didn't. She couldn't write to the topic. *She couldn't understand the question* and couldn't understand when she was and was not writing to the question. Her poor language comprehension was affecting her writing.

We proceeded through the basic V/V process and extended into writing application. In only a few months, Dolores felt she had made enough progress to again try the CBEST test. She took it, but she didn't pass the reading comprehension nor the writing subtest. Disappointed, she took a short break from tutoring, rescheduled the CBEST and then resumed tutoring again. Again only a few months had passed, and again she scheduled to take the CBEST. Although she had once again progressed, her skills were very unstable. She took the test anyway...hoping. But, she didn't pass either section. Now very disappointed and her confidence diminishing, she took a break from tutoring.

Within a few months, determined, she again returned to tutoring. I advised her not to schedule the test until she had worked consistently for at least four months, one hour a day. She was committed to daily reinforcement until her skills stabilized. She worked, more consistently than ever, with an active, assertive, focused clinician. They visualized and verbalized in low level material. Dolores answered interpretive questions. They progressed to dense material, still visualizing and verbalizing interpretively. Dolores wrote, and rewrote, and rewrote again. *She* began to note her writing weaknesses. A few months passed, she took a few weeks off from tutoring, and then took the CBEST. We waited for the results. One day the phone rang. Dolores had just gotten the results in the mail—she passed! She passed both the reading comprehension and writing with more than enough points.

Dolores passed the writing component of the CBEST with a good score due to improvement *first* in her ability to comprehend/think/express and second in her ability to write.

Writing from V/V

Visualizing/Verbalizing can be used as a bridge between oral and written language when the student is ready to construct written paragraphs. *Writing application shouldn't begin until the student is fairly confident and accurate at the sentence-by-sentence level, can confidently process the "main idea" of a paragraph, and give succinct oral summaries.* Here is how to use V/V for writing.

1. *Sentence by sentence imaging/writing*
   After the student has placed a colored square for the sentence and has visualized and verbalized her image, have her number and write a "picture-cue" on a 3X5 card (or smaller). A picture-cue is one word or a few words that trigger the image for a sentence. The cards are numbered and placed on each colored square. For example, in the earlier "Fisher Spider story" that Linda read for the sentence-by-sentence level, the picture-cue cards might look like this:

#1 - brown-black spider, tummy, river.

#2 - spider down plant, water.

#3 - spider fangs, poison, eat.

These picture-cue cards are retrieved after the word summary, placed in order, and used to construct a written paragraph. The student positions and sequences the cards and writes a summary based on the images the picture-cue cards provide. She then edits for the "whole" (generally) and then edits for the specifics with a finger on each word.

2. *Paragraph-by-paragraph imaging/writing*

The above procedure can easily be extended to paragraph-by-paragraph imaging/writing. The picture-cue card represents each paragraph rather than each sentence. The cards are numbered, sequenced, and used to retrieve imaged gestalts for each paragraph. The student uses each picture-cue card as a stimulus for each paragraph. The result is the construction of a written "page summary." She edits her writing, both generally and specifically, and rewrites if necessary.

3. *Grammar and punctuation?*

The V/V program does not formally teach grammar and punctuation. But the imaging/thinking base is used to monitor for grammar and punctuation on the basis that *writing creates images.* Grammar and punctuation *usage* can be determined on the basis of the images created. A comma here or a verb tense there will conjure up specific images.

4. *Expository Writing and Narrative Writing*

When more advanced, students will overlap their imaging/thinking skills from summarizing content to expository and narrative writing. Expository writing serves to inform or explain. Narrative writing is a story or description. *Both narrative and expository writing can use imagery to monitor organization, structure, and punctuation.* See the following section for basic steps in writing instruction.

Basic Steps for Writing Instruction

V/V can be used to assist with written summaries. However, there are additional steps to teaching writing. This section offers a skeletal outline of some basic steps for writing instruction.

Paragraph writing instruction should be in three basic stages: the whole, the parts, and the written paragraph. First develop *thinking/imaging skills and oral language expression;* second teach the *specifics of sentence structure, grammar, and punctuation;* and third the *writing of the paragraph.*

1. *Gestalt thinking and oral language expression*

Gestalt thinking is the foundation for writing and is taught throughout the V/V program. Direct application with the use of picture-cue cards was discussed earlier in this chapter and may be applied at the paragraph writing stage of writing instruction.

2. *Spelling and sentence construction*
Weak spelling can interfere with writing. Individuals with spelling problems describe their frustration about having to write what they can spell rather than what they can think. They often have thoughts that they cannot write down because they have a limited spelling vocabulary. Use the *Auditory Discrimination in Depth Program*, Visual Spelling Chart, and AVW (Analyze, Visualize, Write) technique to teach spelling.

Spelling is a critical part of writing and so is sentence construction. When working with young children, I teach only basic sentence structure and capitalization, periods, and question marks. This is usually easily taught once the child has good oral language expression developed through V/V. If not, the *Fokes Sentence Builder* can be of assistance.

As students get older, their writing becomes more refined and further instruction is necessary. Awareness of sentence structure must be taught: sentence fragments, sentence run-togethers, subject/verb agreement, time/person shift, wordiness, parallel construction, and standard English verbs. Refined punctuation also must be taught: the period, question mark, exclamation mark, semicolon, colon, dash, comma rules, quotation mark, and capital letters. These are effectively discussed and efficiently practiced in a paperback book, *The Least You Should Know About English*. I particularly like this book because it only discusses the *very least* you need to know about English. It is well written (easily understood) and provides practice exercises for each concept. Use it to teach from or to improve your own specifics regarding writing.

3. *Paragraph Writing*
While sentence construction is being taught, overlap to having students copy or edit pre-written paragraphs. The copying and editing tasks familiarize students with the elements of writing before they are asked to construct their own paragraphs. For paragraph copying, simply have the student copy short paragraphs. For paragraph editing, have students edit paragraphs written by other students. Paragraphs can be collected and typed from other students and categorized into editing for spelling, sentence construction, and paragraph organization. When students can successfully edit someone else's paragraph, they will be able to edit their own.

Use V/V to overlap into the actual writing of paragraphs. As presented earlier, paragraph construction is easily initiated and practiced by doing "V/V imaging/writing." By having the student use picture-cue cards, the paragraph organization is already established from the material read and a written summary can easily be constructed. V/V writing prepares the student for constructing her expository or narrative paragraph.

The student will soon begin writing her own paragraph, without the picture-cue cards. This is introduced after students can write a summary paragraph from picture-cue cards, are confident at whole paragraph imaging, and can confidently give oral summaries (word summaries) of a short paragraph. The student reads a paragraph and gives an oral summary and then a written summary without picture-cue cards. When completed, the paragraph is edited generally and specifically, and rewritten if necessary.

After the student constructs a paragraph from her word summary, she must learn to construct a paragraph from scratch! "Free Writing and Clustering" is one way to collect ideas for writing from scratch. Free writing gives the student time to write down any words that come to mind. Spend only a few minutes for this and then choose a word or concept from the free writing and "cluster" by thinking of all the elements of that topic. Encourage imaging for creative thinking. Image the elements that support a concept and then write them down. Number the parts to provide sequence.

By now the student can summarize or create a complete paragraph and is therefore ready to construct a multi-paragraph essay. Begin with V/V paragraph-by-paragraph imaging/writing so that the student is only asked to summarize. The basic elements and structure of a multi-paragraph essay will be provided from the imaged page summary.

Older students may profit from working through some paragraph writing books. *The Least You Should Know About English* and *Structuring Paragraphs* are two books that are very helpful for learning about paragraph structure and extending that structure to essays and reports. *Structuring Paragraphs* also instructs nicely on topic sentence and the general-to-specific paragraph. Use this book either to instruct the student or as a reference for yourself.

Expository Writing

One of the major problems in essay writing is unfocused, non-specific organization. Here is a very helpful formula to force specific writing for an expository thesis. Write a specific topic sentence followed by a sentence with a colon designating two or three areas of specific support for the topic sentence. Discuss each specific from the "colon" second sentence in the body of the thesis and conclude with a summary paragraph. For example:

Paragraph #1

1. Sentence #1: A specific topic sentence.

Jogging is an exercise that can bring back health.

2. Sentence #2: Use a colon and present three reasons that support the topic sentence.

This is due to three specific reasons: 1) increased cardiovascular stimulation, 2) improved muscle tone, and 3) released endorphins to the brain.

Paragraph #2

3. Write supporting details for the first reason: increased cardiovascular stimulation.

Paragraph #3

4. Write supporting details for the second reason: improved muscle tone.

Paragraph #4

5. Write supporting details for the third reason: released endorphins to the brain.

Paragraph #5

6. Write a concluding paragraph that restates the main idea. This is easily mastered if interpretive thinking/comprehension was stimulated with V/V, since drawing conclusions is one of the comprehension skills specifically developed.

The format of topic sentence and supporting details is written in virtually every book on paragraph writing. The *new* element is the very specific second sentence. If high school and college students use a specific second sentence, it will keep their thinking and their writing focused. A similar format can be used for narrative writing.

Narrative Writing

Narrative writing is a description or story. The story will have a setting, main characters, plot, climax, and resolution. This gives a subsequent structure of where, who, problem or action, turning point or climax, and conclusion or resolution. The following narrative formula will give a structure with transition and focus.

Paragraph #1

1. Present the main characters and setting. Write with images in mind and transfer those images to the reader.

Paragraph #2 (or more)

2. Present the plot or action. Number of paragraphs may vary. Again include imagery as foundation for communication.

Paragraph #3 (or more)

3. Present the climax. Number of paragraphs may vary.

Paragraph #4 (final paragraph)

4. Present the conclusion or resolution of plot, action, and climax.

Summary

Visualizing/Verbalizing develops the foundation for writing. "Writing" is easier if thought of as written images. Just as oral language is creating images in the mind of the receiver—*writing is creating images in the mind of the reader.*

If writing is to improve, the student will need to write and edit, write and edit, write and edit. The only way to learn to walk is to walk. The only way to learn to write is to write. Writing is a skill that must be practiced.

Summary of Writing from Visualizing/Verbalizing

step 12

1. Stimulate gestalt processing.
   Develop thinking and oral language comprehension and oral language expression by using the Visualizing/Verbalizing program. This will develop a language base from which writing can be taught.

2. Begin teaching the "parts" for writing.
   Teach sentence structure, basic punctuation, and spelling.

3. Teach paragraph Writing.
   While teaching sentence structure, punctuation, and spelling, overlap to the following:

   a. Paragraph copying.

   b. Paragraph editing—specify if editing for spelling, sentence structure, punctuation, organization, or all of the preceding.

   c. Paragraph summary from V/V image-cue cards. Write and edit.

   d. Paragraph summary without cue cards. Write and edit.

   e. Paragraph summary from scratch—use free writing and clustering.

   f. Page summary with image-cue cards. Write and edit.

   g. Expository paragraphs using specific format for organization and focus. Write and edit.

   h. Narrative paragraphs using specific format for organization and focus. Write and edit.

Part Three

The Summary

The net of reasoning is woven with imagery.

Nanci Bell

Chapter 15

How to Question

Brain processing needs to be stimulated in order for an individual to move from a person who *cannot* image to a person who *can* image. But, telling a "Catherine" to visualize won't *teach* her to visualize.

Questioning from the teacher is the difference between processing and not processing. The questions asked are directly related to the development of imaging and thus are directly related to the development of cognitive processing. A good questioning technique is critical to the V/V process and difficult to learn. We have been taught to tell not to ask.

How to Question?

A good questioning technique embodies these five principles.

1. Avoid yes or no questions

Do not ask questions that require just a yes or no response. Questions such as "Did you picture anything?"… "Does he have…," or… "Will she go to the…" all need only a yes or no response and don't stimulate imaging/thinking. However, if these questions are followed with "what" and "why" they become acceptable.

2. Give choice and contrast

Do ask questions with choice and contrast. Give the student some choices to think with and some contrast within those choices. For example:

"What do you picture the girl wearing—a dress, shorts and a top, or nothing at all?" Note the choices of types of attire and then the contrast of nothing.

What color is the dress—red, pink, blue, polka-dots, stripes?" Again note the choices of color and then some contrast.

"Why did the birds take a bath with dust—to get cleaner, to get dirtier, to just play around...?"

"How does the dust get rid of the bugs—by making them angry, by choking them, making them cough...?"

3. Question to the student's response

Do learn to question to the student's response. When you ask a question and receive a response, use the student's response as the starting place for your next question or stimulus. This allows you to meet the student in his or her thinking—not just your thinking.

If a question is asked and the student gives an unexpected response, should you just ignore it? To the contrary, you should accept each response to promote a climate conducive to interaction. This is not to say that every response is accepted as accurate. But, every response is valued by *acknowledgement. We should have a basic appreciation and respect for the mind of each individual with whom we work—no matter the age or severity of dysfunction.* We can demonstrate respect by acknowledging his response and proceeding to lead the thinking/imaging in the direction of the gestalt.

4. Question to the gestalt

Do question to the imaged gestalt. This is critical and necessitates that *you* be able to discern the gestalt of the information being read or received.

A teacher with an auditory conceptual dysfunction—difficulty perceiving sounds *within* words—cannot develop auditory conceptual processing for her students. The same is true for teaching Visualizing/Verbalizing. The teacher must be able to comprehend language well. She must be able to connect to the gestalt, process the central thought, infer, draw conclusions, and predict. If unable to comprehend and interpret, the teacher will be unable to relevantly question to the imaged gestalt.

If you can judge the gestalt, then direct your questions to that end. You may want to read ahead in a paragraph to know which details to pursue. Although you want to develop detailed imagery, you don't want to develop details that will distract from the gestalt.

Here are sample questions. The text is from Richard Boning's *Specific Skills.*

"In order to trap mustangs, Indians of old waited at the waterhole. At night, when the mustangs came to drink, the Indians waited until the horses were full. Then they would chase after the water-filled mustangs on their own horses."

The gestalt of this paragraph is that the mustangs are difficult to catch, so Indians waited for them to get full of water in order to slow the mustangs down and make it possible to capture them. Which of the following questions leads the student to the gestalt?

Questions #1: "How much water was in the waterhole?" "Was the water dirty or clean?" "Were there rocks in it?"

Questions #2: "What did the horses look like after they drank the water?" "How did their stomach look different?"

Questions #1 will lead the student to image details regarding the water in the waterhole. Is that relevant to the gestalt? Does it matter?

Questions #2 will lead the student to image horses fatter and full of water. Is that a relevant detail toward the gestalt?

It is important to develop detailed imagery but questions #1 ask for irrelevant details, not critical to the gestalt. However, questions #2 ask for imaging that *is* relevant to the gestalt. Visualizing fat, full mustangs leads to visualizing the mustangs as slow and easy to catch.

5. Ask interpretive questions

Do ask interpretive questions. Comprehension is more than just recalling facts. Comprehension is understanding, critical thinking, synthesis, and interpreting. The taxonomy of comprehension skills requires the development of main idea, inference, conclusion, prediction/extension, and evaluation. All of these lead to *reasoning* ability. Because of their significance, let's review interpretive questioning again.

Main Idea Questioning

Questioning for the main idea of a paragraph is introduced at the sentence by sentence level after the student can give fairly confident and accurate picture and word summaries. The main idea can be stimulated by asking the student, "What is the main idea? What did you *see* in each picture (colored square)?"

Soon, the student will only need some prompting with choice and contrast such as, "Was the main idea how mustangs drink water...how Indians get to sleep...how Indians catch mustangs...how mustangs run fast?" Note the inherent contrast in the questions.

Inference Questioning

It can be difficult to ask an inference question. The definition of "infer" will be helpful in knowing what to ask:

1 - *infer:* To conclude from evidence; deduce.
2 - *deduce:* To reach a conclusion by reasoning.

The above definitions establish the necessity of processing the gestalt prior to inferring. We cannot infer adequately from a part, we can only infer from the whole. Therefore, an inference question is asked only after the student can give fairly confident and fluent *word summaries,* and can determine the main idea.

The simplest way to phrase an inference question is to ask *why* or *how,* based on the gestalt. Ask for thinking regarding that which was implied but not directly stated. Here are some examples of questions from the preceding mustang paragraph:

#1: *"Why couldn't Indians catch mustangs without the mustangs being full of water?"* This requires the student to consider that the weight of an Indian will slow down his horse and prevent catching the fast mustang. But, the weight of the water the mustang drinks will slow the mustang down. Then the Indians' horses can run as fast as the mustang...and they finally trap him.

#2: *"Why would Indians need to trap mustangs? Do they eat them?"* This requires the student to consider ideas such as: the Indians need more horses to ride; trapping horses is easier than keeping lots of them in pens and feeding them; there aren't stores around where Indians can buy more horses; and the Indians didn't have automobiles to drive for transportation, etc.

Conclusion Questioning

Again, the imaged gestalt is necessary in order to draw a conclusion. If the student can give succinct word summaries, she will easily be able to draw a conclusion. Initiate the conclusion with, *"From this information we can conclude that... because..."* Give choices with contrast, such as: *"From this information we can conclude that mustangs were slow...or mustangs were fast...or that mustangs drank water only during the day...etc."*

Predict/Extend Questioning

It is easy to ask a predicting/extending question by simply saying, *"From all this information we can predict that..."* or *"What do you think might happen next?"* Give choices and contrast if necessary. Again, the imaged gestalt is a prerequisite. Are you getting it!

Evaluation Questioning

An evaluative question asks the student to evaluate the information with an affective influence. For example, how does the student feel about the information in terms of an opinion, relevancy, and even moral issues.

Summary

Most of us have to learn and practice a good questioning technique.

The five principles for questioning are:

- Do not ask "yes" or "no" questions.
- Question with choice and contrast.
- Respond to the student's response.
- Question to the gestalt.
- Ask interpretive questions.

Learn how to question. The practice is well worth it. I can think of nothing more important to teach than *reasoning*. Stimulating visualizing and verbalizing, and asking interpretive questions from the imaged gestalt, develops comprehension, critical thinking, and reasoning. What a gift when you master it.

Chapter 16

Materials, Levels, Pacing and Practice

As the V/V process unfolded in the preceding chapters, information was sprinkled throughout the pages on suggested materials, grade levels, pacing, and practice. This chapter will offer specifics and clarity—just in case you skimmed a particular section that had an important sprinkle!

Materials

Pictures

The choice of pictures is critical. In the picture to picture stage, the student describes a picture in order to develop the ability to verbalize from a given image. *The picture must be simple.*

When I was discovering this V/V process, I didn't realize how important it would be to choose a simple picture. I chose pictures from magazines or children's books, usually making good choices. However, I soon realized that not everyone made good choices. Often tutors and teachers chose pictures that seemed simple, but weren't. If the picture appeared primary but had lots of detail and background, the student had too much information to describe and the lesson energy evaporated. The student fatigued from too much information to describe and the teacher fatigued from too much information to keep in mind! The lesson was not relevant and wasted time.

The criteria for choosing a picture are:

- One central figure or only a few figures
- Very little detail
- None or very little background
- *Color*

Structure Words
The material for structure words is very simple: 3X5 cards or copy the page in the appendix and have it printed on card stock.

Colored Squares
The colored squares used at sentence by sentence, and paragraph by paragraph, are three-inch squares of different colors. Simply make about 6 to 10 squares. If you don't want to do that, or think you don't have time, use plain 3X5 cards...even paper napkins were used by one parent. I prefer colored *felts* because they are durable, colorful, and an appealing fabric to handle.

Reading Material

The choice of reading material is important. In the initial stages of the V/V process, the material must be short and high in imagery. As the process is more refined, at the whole page and whole chapter levels, the material should be more dense and more abstract.

INITIAL STAGES of V/V: Sentence and paragraph imaging

In the initial stages of V/V, I use Richard Boning's *Specific Skills Series* for high imagery material. This material is widely used and teaches a variety of skills at a variety of grade levels. For example, from first- to twelfth- grade level, the titles are: WORKING WITH SOUNDS, FOLLOWING DIRECTIONS, USING THE CONTEXT, LOCATING THE ANSWER, GETTING THE FACTS, GETTING THE MAIN IDEA, DRAWING CONCLUSIONS, DETECTING THE SEQUENCE.

At the sentence and paragraph imaging stages, use *Getting the Main Idea* and *Drawing Conclusions*. These two books contain short, high imagery, high interest, self-contained paragraphs. They provide an interesting, complete paragraph from which to image and create a gestalt. I seldom use the written question that accompanies each selection. Instead, after the word summary, I generate interpretive questions orally.

FINAL STAGES of V/V: Paragraph by paragraph, page, and chapter noting

Paragraph by paragraph and page imaging require an entire page of context to be visualized and verbalized. It is still important to use high imagery material, so I recommend the following books.

1. Richard Boning, *Specific Skills*: "Getting the Facts," any appropriate level from first through twelfth grade. This contains a full page of interesting, easily imaged material.

2. Richard Boning, *Multiple Skills:* any appropriate level from first through twelfth grade. This is a short page of material with five good comprehension questions, including a main idea and inference.

3. Walter Pauk, *Six Way Paragraphs*: This is eighth through twelfth grade, a short page of material with six good questions on main idea, subject matter, supporting details, conclusions, clarifying devices, and vocabulary in context.

4. Edward Fry, *Reading Drills for Speed and Comprehension*: This book has more than one page of content and should be used for whole page imaging where more content is desired. The readability is seventh through tenth-grade and there are 10 comprehension questions which are broken into two basic groups: recall and interpretive. This book also includes 10 vocabulary questions that I occasionally use where applicable.

5. SAT and GED workbooks have very dense material and good interpretive questions for upper grade students. I urge you to use this material for high school and college students because, as you know, the V/V process is not complete until you have developed interpretive comprehension and critical thinking skills.

6. Schoolbooks are used for chapter noting. The material is content-related such as history, science, health, and English. If working with individuals who are not in school, use subjects of interest and relevancy to their lives.

Grade Level of Written Material

The grade level of the written material is also critical. One of the most serious mistakes made with the V/V process is to choose written material that is too difficult rather than too simple. It is easy to understand why this happens. If working with a sixth-grade boy, it seems that sixth-grade material should be used or even his school work. However, you are not trying to teach any specific material when doing V/V. You are trying to develop imagery, gestalting of information, critical thinking, interpretive thinking, reasoning, recall, and expressive language. Therefore, **begin with low-level material.**

This anecdote will assist you in understanding the importance of choosing the proper grade level of written material. I was working with a community college student named Diana. She was bright but had a moderate to severe comprehension problem for both oral and written language. She was having difficulty passing her college classes and was a poor writer. Her essays and reports were poorly organized, lengthy, and rambling. Her writing was not specific nor focused.

We began V/V to develop her reading comprehension, expressive oral language, written language, etc. She came for 30 minutes of tutoring five days a week and I consulted once a week to guide and pace the treatment. Week after week, I noted that she was not progressing. Every week I gave instructions to continue sentence by sentence imaging in low-level material. But every week, when I checked her imaging and processing, she still was not progressing. I began to question if the tutor was following my plan. He said, "Well, yes...we do sentence by sentence in level D (fourth grade) as you indicated, but...sometimes we don't get to it...or we only do one paragraph because she has homework that she needs to complete. We have spent a lot of time working on her English writing and philosophy."

Philosophy! English! This young woman was unable to create a gestalt from information at the fourth-grade level. She could not give succinct, sequenced oral summaries of low-level information. It would certainly be impossible for us to instruct her in English and philosophy. I then recalled that as I had passed by their sessions, the tutor was doing most of the verbalizing. He cared and was genuinely trying to help her with her most pressing problem—passing her classes. However, he was explaining and reexplaining and she wasn't connecting to his explanations. She was continuing to perform very poorly in her classes and was becoming disenchanted with the tutoring.

I explained again to Diana, *and her tutor*, the importance of working in low-level material with sentence by sentence imagery and insisted that they discontinue any homework tutoring and only work on Visualizing/Verbalizing for the next few weeks. They complied, with reservation, and began sentence by sentence imaging in low level material. Within weeks we moved to higher level material and within a few more weeks Diana noticed that she was automatically imaging *as* she read or listened. She also noticed that she was connecting to the lectures in class, she was beginning to remember what she read in philosophy, her grades spontaneously improved, and *she* began to notice that her writing was rambling and unorganized. Her imaging and verbalizing improved and we moved into higher level material, including her school work. This experience was as fortunate for me as for her—it reinforced for me the *necessity* of working in low-level material to develop imaged gestalts. Working in high-level material too soon is a false economy with little or no return for the time spent.

When using the V/V technique, *you are teaching processing not content*. The goal is to develop an imaged gestalt of content to be recalled and interpreted.

Grade-Level Guidelines

The following guidelines will be helpful for choosing the appropriate level of written material.

1. **Initial sentence by sentence imaging**
    In the initial stages of sentence by sentence imaging, use low-level material, no matter what the age of the student. If the student is in fourth grade or above, begin with third grade. If the student is below third grade, begin with first-grade paragraphs. Since material below third grade is often insipid and without closure, you may wish to slightly modify content as you read to the student. Spice it up just a little but still keep it simple.

2. **Improved sentence by sentence imaging**
    As the student improves at sentence by sentence imaging, move upward through the levels of material. I recommend moving up a grade level when the visualizing and verbalizing is good enough to consider increasing the amount and density of content. How far and how fast you move will depend on the age and grade level of your student, but always begin in low level material and slowly work upward.

3. **Paragraph imaging**
    When you initiate paragraph imaging, you may continue from the grade level of material used in sentence by sentence imaging. However, it is sometimes wise to initially move back a grade level or two, just to lighten the content, and ensure success.

4. **Paragraph by paragraph and page imaging**
    Initiate paragraph by paragraph and page imaging at the same level or go back a level to ensure success. Again, this will lighten content when the student is being asked to connect to more information. Your goal is to move to the student's grade level and potential.

Pacing and Practice

The appendix has a V/V check list for pacing a student. It is self-explanatory and very helpful.

Lessons must have energy and relevancy. Use the following guideline to determine pacing and amount of practice.

1. *Lesson Energy*

The energy and joy in a session is easily diagnosed. If you practice too long on a given step, without forward movement, both you and the student will fatigue. When the lessons are dragging, but the student still needs practice, overlap and extend into the next step. Overlapping and extending will boost the lesson energy, as will having fun—humor.

2. *Lesson Relevancy*

The relevancy of the lesson is a primary concern and requires diagnostic skill. Ask yourself if the lessons are accomplishing the *specific goal* and the *overall goal*. Lesson relevancy requires that you see and accomplish both. Are the lessons accomplishing the goals of each step (specific goal)? Are the lessons accomplishing the goals of the entire Visualizing/Verbalizing process (overall goal)?

If the student has participated in only a week of sentence by sentence imaging, but is already imaging and verbalizing well, move to the next step. The specific goal has been learned—so keep the process going. Don't pursue a certain step just because it seems that the student "shouldn't move that fast." It is not relevant to go over steps that are already mastered. Overlap or move on to the next stage with the reassurance that you can always come back if you have progressed ahead too fast.

Just as it is important not to move too slowly, it is also important not to move too fast simply because you want to get into more difficult material. No matter how relevant you consider the content to be, it will not be relevant if the student can't process it. You won't accomplish the overall goal if you don't teach the student to visualize and verbalize imaged gestalts.

Chapter 17

Clinical and Classroom Management

How to implement the V/V program in the classroom and clinical environment? A classroom environment usually requires working with groups of students, while clinical is usually one-to-one. *Both environments require daily stimulation and diagnostic interpretation of each individual's ability to visualize and verbalize.*

Visualizing/Verbalizing changes and/or develops brain processing. *Remedial V/V must be done five times a week.* It is cognitive training when used preventively and cognitive retraining when used remedially. Stimulation fewer than five times a week results in very slow progress, if any.

Developmental V/V may be done fewer than five times a week, but not less than three times a week. Classrooms implementing the V/V program developmentally note that three times a week is adequate for the majority of students, while students with a severe dysfunction fall into the remedial category and require daily stimulation.

Clinical Management

Remedial V/V
Clinical management is tutorial and simple to organize. For remedial V/V, a daily 60 minute session is recommended in order to allow for enough time to develop *detailed* imagery. Daily thirty minute sessions are the minimum but, one hour a day is preferred remedial V/V because fewer than 60 minutes limits the stimulation. For example, a 30 minute session may only afford enough time to do one or two tasks. The individual just begins to image and the time is up!

Although one hour a day is recommended, the amount of time per session primarily depends on the severity of the dysfunction and the number of days/weeks/months that the student will be able to participate. For example, I have accomplished remedial V/V with college students in one week of intensive tutoring, four hours per day. We were limited to one week since the V/V therapy had to be accomplished during the break between semesters and each of these students had moderate weakness. They made significant gains in comprehension, but would have benefitted from further stimulation, with direct application to their academic requirements.

Developmental V/V

If you are working one-to-one preventively with individuals, developmental V/V may be accomplished in daily 30 minute sessions often for eight to twelve weeks. This is also adequate for remedial V/V if the student has only mild weakness in language comprehension/expression.

Clinical lesson recording and evaluating

It is important to record and evaluate each lesson. This provides the information necessary for the diagnosis of visualizing/verbalizing ability and the assessment of progress. Record the following:

- Note the task (sentence-by-sentence; paragraph imaging; etc.)
- Note the level of material
- Note the mode of receiving the material (receptive, read aloud or silently).
- Evaluate performance per task with one word or short sentence.
- Generalize regarding the amount of questioning or prompting needed.

Here is a sample of a recorded lesson. Record in the following manner rather than a lengthy narrative. The lesson demonstrates the overlap of levels and receiving modes that are possible in a one hour session.

Catherine - a one hour session, after two months of tutoring:
Date: ___   *1. SxS, level D, receptive*
            —images = fair, needs some questioning for details
            —picture summary = good
            —word summary = good
            —main idea = fair
            —inference = OK, if imaged gestalt was strong

            2. SxS, level D, Catherine read aloud
            —images = fair, needs some questioning
            —picture summary = good

—word summary = good
—main idea = good
—inference = good

3. *MS (Multiple Sentence Imaging), Catherine read aloud, level D*
—images = only fair, again need some questioning
—picture summary = good once details imaged for each part,
—word summary = good
—main idea and inference = good

4. *Tried a whole paragraph, receptively to Catherine, level C*
—images = fair but omitted some significant specifics, some gesturing and eye movement.
—had to reread sections in order to image.
—word summary = OK after imaged
—main idea = weak

Classroom Management

The classroom environment usually requires working with groups of children. As stated earlier, the V/V process is cognitive training. This training necessitates on-going diagnosis. The instructor questions toward the imaged gestalt and must note when the student is imaging and not paraphrasing. This is more difficult when working with groups of children, but it can be accomplished. *In the classroom, the V/V program can be administered to individual children, small groups, and the entire class.*

Offer visualizing/verbalizing in individual and small group settings to the children in the most need. Once these students begin to "get" a certain step of the program, the same step can be presented to the entire class. This preface stimulation will give students, that otherwise would have been unable to respond in large group interaction, a head start and success in front of their peers.

Individual Classroom Instruction
Individual instruction can and must be set up in the classroom for the severely impaired child or children in the class. Although there will only be a few children that are severely dysfunctional, they do require one-to-one intervention.

Creativity and determination are necessary to organize for one-to-one interaction. The classroom teacher may be able to provide a daily, fifteen minute one-to-one session with a specific child, and the child's remaining V/V stimulation might be with a group. The teacher may train a parent, peer (cross-age tutor), volunteer (senior citizen), or work experience high school student to do the V/V program, thirty minutes per day, with a specific student. Whichever the case, *the stimulation must be daily.* Severely dysfunctional students will not respond to once or twice a week instruction. *Cognitive retraining requires daily stimulation.*

Daily one-to-one instruction sometimes seems foreign for the classroom teacher to consider. But what is the alternative? If a student is severely dysfunctional, cannot process language receptively or expressively, and is doing very poorly in school and life, is it OK to pass him or her on to the next teacher? Recall what happened to Catherine. After twelve years of school, going from grade to grade, her comprehension was only at a third grade level. Or, is it OK to recommend special classes that also may not address the issue of imagery relevant to comprehension development? Catherine had some form of reading tutoring in the middle grades. Clearly neither scenario is OK. We are educators and we are charged with the responsibility of teaching individuals to think, comprehend, express, and reason.

Small Group Classroom Instruction
Small group instruction in V/V works well for those children in the classroom that have a moderate dysfunction. The stimulation should be daily. For example, implement the V/V program in place of reading comprehension stimulation for a few months. But, where is reading comprehension instruction in the classroom? In consulting with numerous school districts, and talking with administrators and teachers, I have concluded that we frequently don't find daily comprehension instruction in the curriculum. Unbelievable. It seems that often instruction in comprehension is assigning written questions to be answered—*testing not teaching comprehension.*

Children progress through the grades, unable to comprehend language. Yet, what better skill could we teach a child? Is it better to teach science and history and English rather than language comprehension? If we teach language comprehension and decoding, children can and will teach themselves science, history, and English.

Then where to put V/V in the curriculum? Without asking teachers to add to an already crowded day, the best choice is either in the reading or the language time. Keep in mind, if V/V is done daily, it will not have to be done the entire school year. Small group instruction might only be necessary for a few months and then developmental V/V can be continued with the entire class a couple of times a week —perhaps right after lunch during the storytime.

Small group instruction requires some modest manipulation of the V/V steps. These modifications are summarized on the next page and on the appropriate summary page for each step.

1. *Picture-to-Picture*
   The teacher has each student take turns describing a given picture and reverbalizing through the structure words. Viewing the group as a collective student makes it easy to implement the procedures.

2. *Word Imaging*
   The teacher has each student take turns visualizing and verbalizing a collective image and reverbalizing through the structure words. The teacher is responsible for imaging, questioning, and summarizing.

3. *Sentence by Sentence and Multiple Sentence Imaging*
   The teacher has each student take turns visualizing and verbalizing a sentence. For example, Hank may V/V the first sentence, Alice the second, Willard the third; then Hank reverbalizes the structure words, Joe gives a picture summary, and Hazel gives the word summary. In this way all students participate in the same paragraph. When extending to higher order thinking skills, each student answers a question.

4. *Paragraph Imaging*
   The teacher has each student read or receive an entire paragraph, give a word summary, and respond to oral interpretive comprehension questions.

5. *Paragraph-by-Paragraph Imaging*
   The teacher has each student read or receive one paragraph, place a colored square per paragraph, and give a paragraph word summary. For example, Hank reads the first paragraph, gives a word summary, and interprets. Hazel reads the second paragraph, gives a word summary, and interprets. Willard reads the third paragraph, etc. The teacher and other students may question to check for imaging. Interpretive questions are answered and then one student gives a page summary.

6. *Page Imaging*
   The teacher has each student read an entire page, orally or silently, discuss images, give a page summary, and answer oral or written interpretive questions. If each student reads the page silently, visualizing and verbalizing can be used to compare interpretation of the page and keep students actively participating.

The most difficult part of group instruction is diagnosing whether each student is developing gestalt imaging or just chiming in with the other students. Questioning provides an answer. If the student cannot verbalize his image with detail, then visualization may be in doubt. Observe him for eyes up or "defocused," as well as gesturing and spontaneous responses to print and the images of others.

Large Group Instruction
Large group instruction is done with the entire class and basically uses the same modifications as small group instruction, except that each student may not have a turn and the teacher will be at the front of the class.

The teacher may use a flannel board for the colored squares—felts. For example, as the sentence by sentence step is practiced, the teacher might choose different students to V/V each sentence. The student places a felt on the flannel board and verbalizes an image. The class can participate by asking questions for detailed images. When the paragraph is complete, different students may be chosen to give a picture and word summary.

Imaging with the entire class presents the same diagnostic challenge as described earlier, but it also presents a new challenge. Specific images will be somewhat different for each child. Although this is true, don't let the students be overly concerned if Hank's image is slightly different from Hazel's. Remember, *the specifics may be somewhat different, but the gestalt will be the same.* The teacher should allow for some specific differences within the images, but emphasize and stimulate the sameness of the gestalt.

When working with the entire group, it is helpful to have a technique for managing the students. I observed Peg Klotz, a classroom teacher, work with her entire class and have the attention and active participation of each student. She used pre-arranged signals with her class so students wouldn't have to flail their arms or shout out answers, yet still be rapt with attention. The specific signals were:

1. She said "think" and touched her head which meant "think" not "say" and not raise hands. Then she identified a student to respond to the stimulus. Note, that she identified a specific student *after* (not before) she said "think." By doing this she had the entire class thinking and anticipating, since she might call on anyone.
2. If wanting the entire group to respond orally, she opened her arms to them, palms up.
3. She *invited* students to raise their hands if they knew the answer.

Group instruction can be productive and progress can be achieved by noting and accommodating to overcome the inherent difficulties. Doing V/V daily in a group —while diagnosing for visualizing and verbalizing, questioning to develop the imaged gestalt, and stimulating interpretive comprehension and thinking— improves language comprehension and expression. It is worth it.

Chapter 18

Additional
Concerns and Questions Answered

I feel as though I haven't left this keyboard in years... I am looking quite haggard, fatigued, and am anxious to complete this compilation of thoughts. However, there are additional concerns and questions that require attention, but not separate chapters, before this book can be completed.

Vocabulary

Can weak oral vocabulary impede the imaging process? Certainly. When an individual is receiving or reading language, and thereby imaging the concept, she must be able to understand—image—the meaning of the words used to present the concept. Obviously, if the she doesn't understand the meaning of a particular word, she can't conjure up an image for the concept presented. For example, if Hazel is reading the sentence, "...two or three *sentries* position themselves on...," and if she doesn't have images for "sentries," then she will be unable to visualize the content and concept presented. If Hank is reading a sentence and doesn't know the meaning of the word "funeral," then he also doesn't have the imagery base to visualize the content containing that word. It is a sign that Hank and Hazel are beginning to self-correct, and image automatically, when they *question vocabulary*. If Hazel stops reading, asks for the meaning of sentries, looks puzzled, or reads on to try to determine vocabulary by imaging the remaining context—she is *expecting* to connect to print. However, students with a language comprehension dysfunction often create a different scenario. They continue reading words *without expecting to get meaning*. They don't question vocabulary since they are not expecting to connect to language anyhow.

But, vocabulary can be developed with imagery. I often put "vocab words" on 3X5 cards. The front of the card has the vocabulary word and the back of the card has the student's picture-cue *and the word used in a sentence*.

Although, dictionaries were meant to assist with vocabulary development, many students with weak vocabularies and weak language comprehension may not experience success when using them. They often cannot understand (image) the written definition. Also, they often have difficulty understanding grammar which makes it useless for word-meaning to be explained in terms of grammatical usage, such as the designation of a word as a noun, verb, or adjective. Although problematic, dictionaries are necessary, so select a dictionary that not only gives the definition but also *uses the word in a sentence*. The latter assists the student with imaging the meaning, and understanding the usage of the word. Not all dictionaries use the word in context, so choose one carefully. Note the difference in clarity between these dictionary definitions:

From Funk & Wagnalls Standard Encyclopedic Dictionary

volatile - *adj.* 1. Evaporating rapidly at ordinary temperatures on exposure to the air. 2. Capable of being vaporized. 3. Easily influenced; changeable. 4. Transient, ephemeral.

From Thorndike Barnhart Junior Dictionary (now Scott Foresman)

volatile - 1. evaporating rapidly; passing off readily in the form of vapor: *Gasoline is volatile.* 2. light and changeable in spirits: *Pat has a volatile disposition. Adj.*

A dictionary that places words in context does help create images for word-meaning; however, individuals cannot memorize all the words in a dictionary. A resource of vocabulary words appropriate for different grade levels is needed. The following are some books written specifically for vocabulary development.

1. *Teaching Vocabulary*, LinguiSystems Inc., 716 17th Street, Moline Il., 61265. There are two volumes: Volume 1 Grades K-4 and Volume 2 Grades 5-8. The words are defined, compared with semantically same/different words, and used in context.

2. *EDL Word Clues*, Educational Developmental Laboratories, Inc., A Division of McGraw-Hill, Huntington, New York. *Word Clues* was written in the 1960's and is a programmed text that presents vocabulary in context and then provides lessons that give experience deducing meaning from text. There are separate books for each grade level, from elementary to very advanced.

3. *Vocabulary Drills*, Edward B. Fry, Jamestown Publishers, P.O. Box 9168, Providence, Rhode Island 02940. Numerous vocabulary words are presented in the context of a few paragraphs of text. The student is asked

to deduce word-meaning from context and then presented with numerous reinforcement tasks such as analogies, antonyms, synonyms, and multiple choice questions for definition. There are two levels: Middle Level Grades 6-8 and Advanced Level Grades 9-12.

Once the individual becomes a "reader," vocabulary can be expected to develop spontaneously. As Hazel reads—and enjoys reading—new vocabulary will be discerned by her imaging/comprehending mind.

Television, Radio Shows, Tapes/Records, Poetry

I have been asked many times if television has had an effect on reading comprehension and imaging. The answer is yes. The book *Endangered Minds: Why Our Children Don't Think*, Healy, 1990, concurs emphatically. The interference from television is two-fold: television creates the images for the brain and large quantities of time are spent "watching" television.

The first issue is obvious—television makes the images for our brain. The part of the brain that creates images is probably not as active when absorbing the images emanating from the television set. Consider the difference between television and old-time radio. As a child I listened to a few of the radio dramas and still have vivid images of the characters and settings. Not only was my brain creating images from the absorption of language, but the radio show enhanced my imagery with sound effects. Roy Rogers and Dale Evans riding their horses along, singing "Happy Trails to You," and Gildersleeve thumping around the house and community—are images still filed somewhere in my brain.

Second, television is avidly viewed by many children. Hours and hours of television time are spent daily as individual brains are developing. With television we don't have to image. We don't have to exchange language. We don't have to interact with language. This is not to say that television lacks benefits. Television, as well as movies, can be a positive learning experience in that children can vicariously experience and learn about things they might otherwise not have an opportunity to learn, such as other cultures, nature, animals. *It is the amount of television time that interferes with language comprehension/expression.*

I also consumed hours of stories and story-record time as a child. I listened and lived with Cinderella, Snow White, Robin Hood, Little Toot, and I had a mother who read aloud to me—all which developed imagery. I recommend the *Read-Aloud Handbook,* by Jim Trelease, for inspiring reading. He eloquently evidences the benefits of reading aloud to children and provides a detailed guide of 300 read-aloud books.

Imagery from language can be stimulated by using cassette tapes of old-time radio shows or children's stories. These can just be enjoyed or actually used as part of the V/V program. For example, if you purchase a story-tape with a picture-book, get rid of the book and create your own images. Stop the tape at any appropriate amount of stimuli, visualize and verbalize, and ask interpretive questions.

Poetry also can be an excellent source of language to image. Poetry inspires imagery.

The Rabbit
When they said the time to hide was mine,
I hid back under a thick grape vine.

And while I was still for the time to pass
A little gray thing came out of the grass.

He hopped his way through the melon bed
And sat down close by a cabbage head.

He sat down close where I could see,
And his big still eyes looked hard at me.

His big eyes bursting out of the rim,
And I looked back very hard at him.

Elizabeth Madox Roberts, From *The Golden Treasury of Poetry*

Night
The sun descending in the west,
The evening star does shine;
The birds resilient in their nest,
And I must seek for mine.
The moon like a flower
In heaven's high bower,
With silent delight
Sits and smiles on the night.

Farewell green fields and happy groves,
Where flocks have took delight.
Where lambs have nibbled, silent moves
The feet of angels bright;
Unseen they pour blessing
And joy without ceasing,
On each bud and blossom,
And each sleeping bosom.

They look in every thoughtless nest,
Where birds are covered warm;
They visit caves of every beast,
To keep them all from harm.
If they see any weeping
That should have been sleeping,
They pour sleep on their head,
And sit down by their bed.

William Blake, from *The Golden Treasury of Poetry*

Poetry, story-records, story-tapes, and books are good sources of language from which to visualize and verbalize. However, they are not usable if the individual can't image. If Hazel has difficulty imaging/comprehending language, then reading aloud to her, or letting her listen to a story-tape won't benefit her. She'll be bored or fatigued while you on the other hand are raptly engrossed in the content! Many parents of children with language comprehension weakness indicate that they read aloud to their child, but he or she didn't enjoy it. Wiggles and boredom soon ensued as the story progressed. The same is true in the classroom. Many teachers have included a read-aloud storytime after lunch, only to find that some children can't attend. These children also often exhibit behavior problems or learning difficulty.

Auditory Memory and Oral Directions

Auditory memory for sentences and the ability to follow oral directions are likewise affected by weak imaging. Students with a severe language comprehension dysfunction may not remember what has been said to them nor follow oral directions. The language connects only in a few "parts." For example, I completed a diagnostic evaluation on a young man named John. He graduated from high school but his grades were poor and he tried one semester at a community college, only to fail. His oral language comprehension was very weak and his reading comprehension became unstable at the third grade level, placing him at the *13th* percentile. He could not easily image when he read. He also couldn't follow oral directions on the job or at home. He worked on his family farm with a kind and intelligent father as his "boss." His father said, "If John is given more than one direction at a time, he is unable to follow even simple instructions." Indeed, diagnostic testing placed John at a six-year-old mental age level in following oral directions.

Once able to visualize and verbalize from oral and written material, John was able to connect to language *as* it entered the brain. He *automatically* visualized oral directions given to him. To insure the application of V/V to directions, we included oral directions to be imaged. When given multiple oral directions, he *expected* to image and connect, and he learned to ask for a direction to be repeated, if necessary, in order to visualize. John progressed to a functional level and had a skill available to assist him with remembering.

Images are too Detailed

There is a certain type of student that tends to include too much detail in his or her imagery. This student is usually "talkative" but tends to be verbally unfocused. Although it is important to stimulate imagery, the *excessive imaged detail departs from the relevancy of the expressed thought or content*. The images tend to spill into areas of irrelevancy and either lose or muddy the gestalt. Therefore, instead of probing for details, *restrain excessive images and direct to the relevancy of the gestalt*.

For example, you might put out three 3X5 cards which you have *illustrated* for the concepts of *not enough, just right*, and *too much* detail. After verbalizing, the student points to the card which best describes his analysis of how much detail he included in his verbalization. The teacher gives feedback. Obviously, this is also effective for the student that doesn't give enough detail.

Eyes that Note Imaging

I have mentioned that imaging can be determined by movement of the eyes. Eyes that *defocus or go up* are an indication that visualizing is in progress. My awareness of this came from a workshop on NLP, Neuro Linguistic Programming. I recommend you read more about NLP in *The Structuring of Magic* books and *Frogs to Princes*.

It is no accident that students with a severe language comprehension dysfunction don't have eye movements that note imaging and they also don't take their eyes from the face of the teacher/tutor. The first time I noticed this phenomenon was while working with a young man of Vietnamese descent. He had been in the United States since a very young boy and had a severe language comprehension/thinking problem. In going through the V/V process, he almost never took his eyes from my face. He stared and stared at me, even when he was trying to gesture and image. I kept waiting for his eyes to indicate visualization, but they just stayed on my face. I finally indicated to the clinician working with him that we would not let him look at her during the time we wanted him to visualize. She wouldn't watch him and he wouldn't watch her.

This was not an isolated case. I have noticed that individuals of all ages, with a severe dysfunction in comprehending language, have this same phenomenon of watching the teacher intently...staring. I believe they are doing this partly from fear of being wrong and partly because they need verification and validation from the face of another individual. They have little confidence in *their* own thinking and correctness. Since they connect to only parts of what they hear or read, they have been in many situations where they appeared foolish, weren't able to comprehend conversation, weren't able to comprehend written material, weren't able to pass a test, and weren't able to "get" what was going on around them. They readily noted their lack of "intelligence" based on the feedback from their peers, teachers, and parents. It is not surprising that they needed to read a face for validation of their worth.

Time Line

Imaging content often requires imaging an era or period in history. But, many individuals with language comprehension weakness don't appear to have images for periods of history and don't have a "time line" of history in mind. They have no or little perspective of history—no gestalt. They can't image details for the 1800's, 1700's, Middle Ages, Romans, etc., and cannot place eras in relation to one another and the gestalt of history. The "Romans" and "World War II" are all the same—the past. I am including the following general time line as a representation of some major events in history. You may need to create your own, show movies of specific eras, and get books with pictorial representations to assist individuals in imaging the perspective of history.

General Time Line for Western Civilization

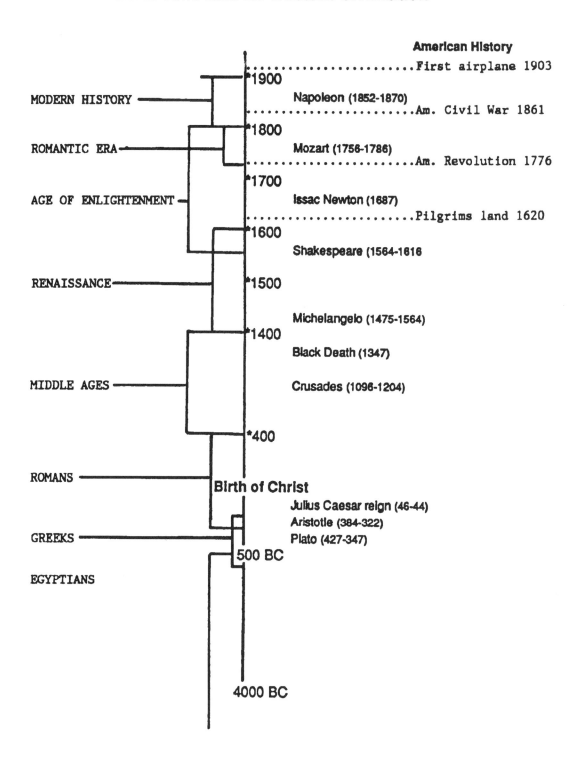

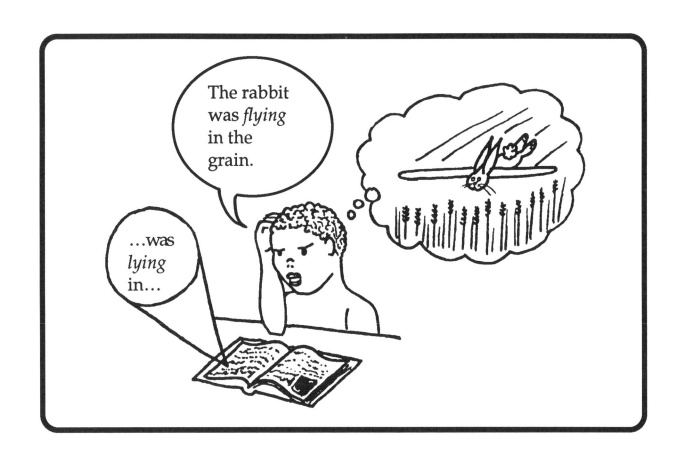

or...

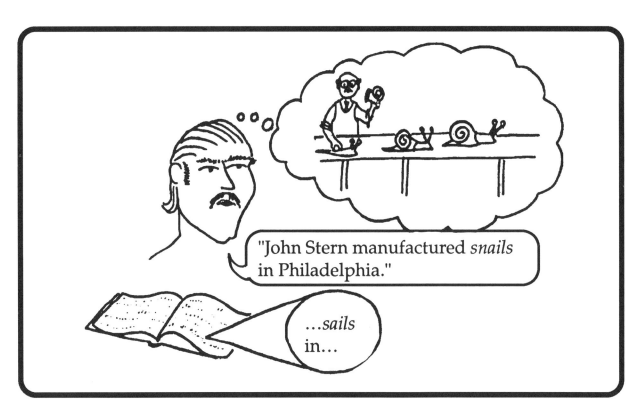

Chapter 19

The Circles and the Reading Process

I cannot leave this encounter with you without discussing my *circles* and my favorite topic of the reading process. Reading is the one area in school that cuts across all other areas. Reading is critical to science, social studies, health, English, etc. Therefore, the reading process gets an entire chapter of specific discussion and analysis. First, it is important to recognize that ***the only reason to read is to get meaning from print.*** From that premise we can proceed. What are the elements of the *process* underlying what we term reading?

For many years the various camps in the discipline of reading have disputed the critical aspects of reading. These disputes could even be likened to religious wars. Some professionals advocate primarily teaching *phonics*. Some advocate primarily teaching a *look-say* approach for the sight recognition of words. Some don't teach phonics and place very little emphasis on teaching the recognition of words. Instead, they advocate teaching the use of *context cues* with a "guessing" strategy. These camps debate whether phonics should be taught or not taught. Or they debate which is more important—phonics or context cues. Or they debate which is more important—phonics or sight words.

The reading camps have been correct concerning the *critical* elements of the reading process. Phonics, sight words, and contextual constraints are necessary ingredients in the *process* of reading. However, not just one element is critical—all are critical for independent reading skill. *Reading is a complex integration of processes, with comprehension the concluding process.*

The reading process requires the integration of four primary functions: 1) phonetic processing, 2) sight word recognition, 3) contextual constraints/oral vocabulary, and 4) imagery for comprehension. The first three parts are labeled auditory, visual, and language—and shown in three circles. The fourth and most critical part is comprehension. The following diagram presents my paradigm of the reading process.

Reading Circles Diagram

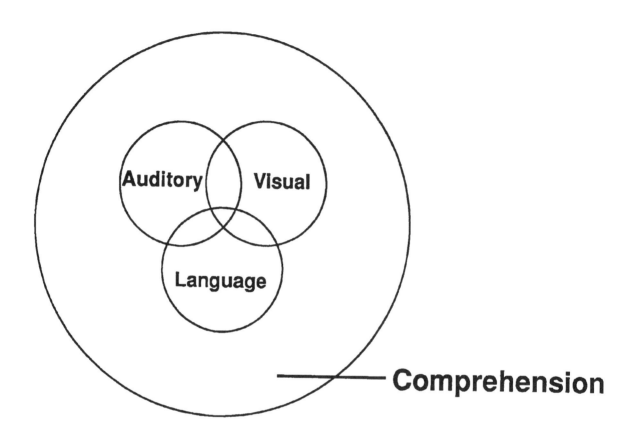

In the diagram above:

1. *The auditory circle represents phonetic processing.* This is not "spit and grunt" phonics, but confident and accurate word attack skills. The ability to *sound out* a word, accurately and fluently, is critical because we cannot memorize all the words in the English language. Good readers—decoders—have good word attack skills.

2. *The visual circle represents sight word recognition.* This is the ability to recognize a base of words instantly, without the need for phonetic processing. It is critical to have a well-established sight word base or we would have to phonetically process each word as we read. Hence, slow, laborious contextual reading.

3. *The language circle represents vocabulary and use of context.* This is the ability to understand the meaning of isolated words orally and use context cues based on the semantics (meaning) and syntax (grammar) of the

written material. We can anticipate words based on context. Good readers have this ability. *This circle does not represent comprehension.*

The Auditory Circle

Auditory processing is a critical function in the process we have termed reading. It is the ability to sound out words based on their individual sounds. We term this ability *word attack*. It is only logical that phonetic processing is a necessary ingredient in the reading process. It is not possible to memorize all the words in the English language nor is it possible to accurately guess at all of them based on contextual cues. It is important to decode accurately since decoding errors can change imagery and thus change comprehension.

In the extreme, years ago, the linguists preached that all one needed to be a good reader was the ability to phonetically process words. Rudolph Flesch wrote in his book, *Why Johnny Can't Read,* that America's reading problems would be solved if only schools taught more phonics. The teaching of reading became enamored with phonics instruction and minimized the importance of getting meaning from print. Some linguistic reading series were produced that taught students to phonetically process words without concern for comprehension of the content. Comprehension was *assumed*.

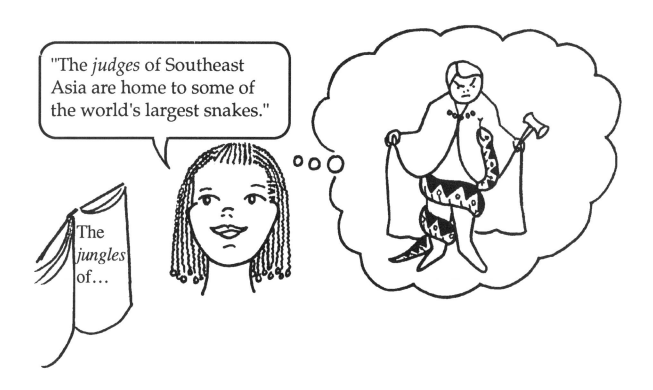

Phonetic processing is not the only element in the reading process, but *it is critical to reading*. Unfortunately, at least a third of our population cannot respond to phonics instruction. These individuals can usually learn sound/letter associations in isolation, such as P = /p/, T = /t/, K = /k/. But, they have an auditory conceptual dysfunction and cannot perceive those same sounds when they come in a syllable—a word. Usually bright, these individuals *cannot perceive the NUMBER of sounds in a syllable, the IDENTITY of the sounds in a syllable, or the ORDER of sounds in a syllable.* Therefore, though they have been taught phonics, they might look at the word *"stream"* and say *"steam."* They might look at *"immigration"* and say *"imagination."* They cannot auditorily judge their error. They also might spell *gril* for *"girl,"* *eqetment* for *"equipment,"* or make speech errors such as *"baf"* for *"bath," "subduce"* for *"seduce."* All these errors—in reading, spelling, and speech—are examples of what is termed *auditory conceptualization dysfunction.* Simply stated, *individuals with an auditory conceptual dysfunction cannot perceive sounds within words.*

The issue of auditory conceptualization deserves much space here due to the critical relationship between decoding skills and auditory conceptual processing. Both educators and laymen have found it difficult to understand an auditory conceptualization dysfunction. Parents and teachers have asked, "Does it mean that the students don't hear well?" The answer is *no,* usually the students hear the whole word very well. Auditory acuity is usually not impaired. The impairment instead is in not being able to perceive each of the sounds that are in a syllable/word. Individuals cannot auditorily segment the word into "parts." They perceive the "whole" of the word but not the separate "parts." This is the exact reverse of individuals with a language comprehension dysfunction, who perceive a few "parts" but not the "whole." Interesting.

As one would expect, individuals with this specific auditory conceptual dysfunction have difficulty decoding words. They usually track the initial or final sounds in a word but the interiors of words scramble or wash for them—auditorily not visually. For example, when Johnny looks at *"stream"* and says *"steam,"* he *sees* each letter correctly but he does not perceive that he has omitted the /r/ sound. His teacher or parent may even point to the letter *r* and ask what letter he sees and what sound it makes. He verifies accurate visual processing by noting that he sees the letter *r* and he also knows the sound of it—then reads the word again as *"steam."* Although surprising to many people, Johnny did see the letter **r** and he knew the sound...and he thought he included it when he said *"steam."* His auditory system didn't monitor, especially in the interior part of the word, whether what he said matched what he saw.

An auditory conceptual dysfunction would be diagrammed as:

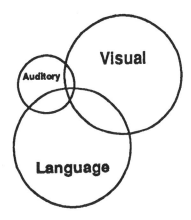

Individuals of all ages and backgrounds may have an auditory conceptual dysfunction which impairs their ability to decode words. The treatment to develop auditory conceptualization focuses on another modality to support and ultimately develop auditory segmentation. This modality is the source of sounds—*the mouth*. Individuals can be taught to perceive sounds by *experiencing* the motor movement of those sounds. This procedure begins with isolated sounds—consonants and vowels—and moves to the syllable and multisyllable level. Moving through a series of specific steps, all students of all ages can develop their auditory conceptualization, thereby developing their word attack and decoding skills. In using the Lindamood®*Auditory Discrimination in Depth (ADD) Program*, I have had significant success with every student and have seen dyslexic adults gain two to four years in decoding skills in one to six months of auditory conceptual tutoring.

In summary, the auditory circle is critical to the reading process but not possible without well-developed auditory conceptual processing.

The Visual Circle

The visual circle represents the ability to recognize a large base of words instantly. This is the sight recognition of words, without phonetic processing. Years ago this type of reading instruction was termed the *Look-Say* method. Words were simply flashed to students, over and over, until they were recognized and remembered. When the Look-Say method was implemented fully, no phonetics were taught. Many individuals today still lament that they were not taught phonics just because they happened to be caught in that particular period of our educational history.

The visual circle is not addressing visual tracking or visual perception. Students with poor visual perception can still be excellent decoders and comprehenders. Although weak visual tracking may interrupt fluency, neither of these is a *primary* contributor to the reading process.

When an individual has weak auditory processing and thus weak decoding skills, he has to attempt to compensate by memorizing massive amounts of words. For example, at the Lindamood-Bell Learning Processes Center we worked with a neurosurgeon who had a severe dysfunction in auditory conceptualization. His spelling was very weak and he recounted having to memorize hoards of medical terminology for both reading and spelling. He worked hours and hours memorizing words based on their orthography, not their sounds. He did manage to compensate—memorize lots of words—better than most people, but he never managed to compensate completely. He resisted reading orally because people laughed at his mispronunciations. He had written numerous medical papers that he never presented orally because of his insecurity with oral reading.

Sight word recognition is an important element in the reading process. Without the ability to quickly and accurately recognize words by sight, the individual would have to phonetically process each word and/or guess from context. Both of which may impair reading rate and comprehension.

The Language Circle

The language circle represents both oral vocabulary and the use of contextual cues. The reading process requires a good oral vocabulary to understand the meaning of each word that is decoded and also requires the ability to anticipate content from context cues.

The use of contextual cues is currently a popular reading strategy. Psycholinguists feel the use of context to be the most crucial strategy to independence and comprehension in reading. They believe that reading words is not a critical element in the reading process and that the major emphasis in reading instruction should be on developing the language background and ability to hypothesize (guess) at a word based on the context of the material. In pure form they do not believe in teaching phonics or sight words. They expect students to anticipate context based on the students' language experience and background. In other words, Johnny is to guess at words based on the semantics (meaning) or syntax (grammar) of the sentence.

Many individuals, such as Catherine, can anticipate context in sentences. Catherine could self-correct based on the syntax and semantics of sentences not the overall content of the paragraphs. She still couldn't comprehend.

Good readers can anticipate context, but what of poor readers? Can poor readers use context cues? It is true that for many poor readers, their primary reading strategy is to guess at or skip words—use context cues. However, it is also true that many poor readers are also not able to hypothesize accurately from context *because they cannot decode enough words to wager a good guess.* For example, if they can only read a few words in a sentence they won't be able to guess at the other words and get meaning. Or, they may have numerous decoding errors that cause them to hypothesize inaccurately the next word or words. Often their word-guess fits both the semantics and syntax of the sentence, but is not the correct word and thus interferes with imagery and comprehension.

It is important to remember that although good readers do anticipate context, good readers also have well developed word attack and word recognition skills. Poor readers do not and the use of context cues is often the only strategy available to them. Unfortunately their reading level depends on knowing enough words to guess at the other words. Very bright individuals may read years below their potential because a memorized sight vocabulary and the use of context cues are the only reading strategies available to them. I have met, diagnosed, and remediated many high school, college, and adult dyslexics who read at the third- and fourth-grade level because they have weak auditory processing and have compensated to the maximum level with visual memory and context.

The language circle is a critical element in the reading process but it does not guarantee comprehension. Reading is an integration of processes and all the circles must be developed to be a good reader.

Comprehension

In the first years of my clinical experience, I believed that when I had developed all three areas of auditory, visual, and language in the reading process, the student would be an independent reader. I was accurate in that the student would be an independent decoder, but not necessarily an independent reader. *The most critical element in the reading process is the ability to connect to and comprehend language.*

The comprehension circle surrounds the other three circles to illustrate the significance of meaning. It cannot be considered just a part of the language circle. It is separate and significant. As the previous chapters in this book have discussed, there are many individuals who can read the words well—have the three circles well developed—but cannot comprehend or get meaning from what they have read. The outer circle, of fully connecting to print through images, is not available to them. When they read, the information goes in one ear and out the other, with just a few parts recalled. They don't process a gestalt, and consequently have no base for interpretive comprehension and critical thinking. It is my hypothesis that visualizing is the basis for language comprehension. Since this entire book has been devoted to discussing the comprehension circle, nothing further will be said here.

Classification of Reading Disorders

Once we understand the process involved in reading, we can *classify* reading disorders and remediate accordingly.

The only reason to read is to get meaning from print and mouthing sounds is useless, of course. Any interference with comprehension is a reading disorder. There are three *primary* types of reading disorders:

- Decoding disorder
- Language comprehension disorder
- Combination of a decoding and a comprehension disorder

Decoding Disorder
A "decoding disorder" means that the individual has weakness in word recognition and word attack, and/or oral vocabulary preventing understanding of each decoded word. One or all the three circles may not be well developed, but usually the primary weakness is in the auditory circle.

Individuals with a decoding disorder are usually classified as dyslexic—reading below their oral language potential. They cannot decode words accurately. They may look at *"was"* and say *"saw,"* *"brook"* and say *"book,"* *"destroy"* and say *"destory,"* *"malignant"* and say *"malijent,"* *"marriage"* and say *"margin,"* etc. A decoding disorder interferes with comprehension of content because individuals cannot accurately read enough words to process the content.

I have observed an interesting phenomenon, alluded to previously. Individuals with a decoding disorder frequently don't have a language comprehension disorder. They *are* able to connect to language and have *good comprehension if they can read enough of the significant words in the text.* I have noted both children and adults struggling with decoding the words, but able to comprehend well at the completion of a paragraph. They don't have the comprehension problem of not connecting to language. If they have comprehension difficulty, it is only the result of poor decoding, not *poor* imaging/language connection.

An individual with a decoding disorder also may have good listening comprehension and good vocabulary, but poor decoding skills, and poor auditory conceptualization for sounds within words. As stated earlier, although other areas may be weak, the *primary* weakness is usually in auditory segmentation. These individuals cannot judge sounds within words and therefore cannot judge if what they say matches what they see. This affects comprehension.

Decoding and Comprehension Disorder
Another common type of reading disorder is a combination of both a *decoding disorder* and a *language comprehension disorder*. Readers who have weaknesses in both areas can neither decode well nor comprehend well. Their disability may be more severe in one area than the other. For example, they may have a severe dysfunction in auditory conceptualization and thus a severe dysfunction in decoding, but only a moderate dysfunction in comprehension, or vice versa. *The focus of treatment should be on the primary weakness and both areas should be developed.*

Comprehension Disorder
Disability and weakness in language comprehension is the focus of this book. A "comprehension disorder" is when the individual reads the words well but with no connection. These individuals often use semantic and syntactic cues *for each sentence.* They may self-correct from context, read sentences with some expression, and ultimately make few decoding errors, but when they complete the paragraph, they remember only a few details and *have no gestalt. The words went in accurately but didn't connect from sentence to sentence.* These individuals may have good word recognition, good word attack, good auditory conceptualization for sounds in syllables, and good oral vocabulary, but weak oral language comprehension, weak reading comprehension, and weak oral/written language expression.

We do not usually term these individuals "dyslexic" since they can decode the words well. Nor has there been room for them in special reading classes, since the classes are filled with decoding disorders. Yet, a *language comprehension disorder* may be more debilitating than a decoding disorder because the comprehension problem is usually in both written and oral language. This means that these individuals have difficulty understanding and interpreting not only what they read, but also what they hear. The oral language disability, even if moderate, affects their entire lives, not just while they are reading. They may be impaired in their ability to understand and interpret movies, lectures, conversation, and any area of life that requires language comprehension and expression.

In my opinion, we are just becoming aware of the seriousness and extent the of this comprehension/critical thinking problem. I am clearly not alone in this assessment. Current research and testing suggests a serious downward trend in higher-order comprehension and critical thinking skills. Recent scores from the National Assessment of Educational Progress (NAEP) show specific deficiencies in what they term higher-order reasoning skills, including those necessary for advanced reading comprehension, math and science. Despite efforts to strengthen elementary and high school curriculums students of all ability levels are showing virtually no gains in higher-order thinking skills, NAEP (1987). "The effects of these universally noted trends have begun to show up even in highly selective colleges, as professors find they must water down both reading and writing assignments as well as expectations for analytic reasoning," Healy (1990).

"Young students may be sounding out the words better, but they are actually understanding less," (1988). Children cannot comprehend, remember, and apply what is read. The 1986 NAEP report found, as have other recent assessments, that students' related problems in reading and expressing ideas in writing stem mainly from difficulty with verbal reasoning, Healy (1990).

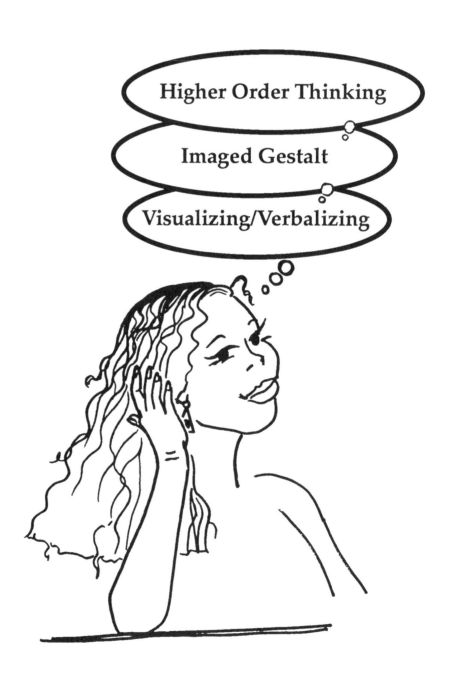

Chapter 20

The Brain Sees

T*he brain sees* in order to store and process information. If we are comprehending, we are imaging the concepts. If we are processing sounds, we are imaging the letters. If we are thinking, we are subtly imaging. This *seeing* is very rapid, very automatic, and very assumed by those that do it well.

That the brain sees is also interestingly discussed in the book, <u>Fire in the Crucible: The Alchemy of Creative Genius</u>. Briggs (1988) examined the reccurring experiences of the greatest creative minds of all times and the mental strategies and tactics they employed when they worked. Their *genius* had to do with *vision*.

"Mozart said that a piece would grow in him until 'the whole, though it be long, stands almost complete and finished in my mind, so that I can survey it, like a fine picture or a beautiful statue, at a glance. Nor do I hear in my imagination the parts successively, but I hear them, as it were, all at once.'

Praised for one of his poems, Shelley said that the words conveyed only a shadow of what he saw. Beethoven wrote of being inspired by the contemplation of the night sky, but that 'when from time to time I try to give shape and form in sound to the feelings aroused within me, alas! I meet with cruel disappointment. In disgust I throw away the sheet of paper I have soiled, and am almost convinced that no earthborn being can ever hope to set down by means of sounds, words, colour, or in sculpture, the heavenly pictures that rise before his awakened imagination!'

Sculptor Auguste Rodin said he was able to represent different parts of the body by visualizing the interior volumes: 'I forced myself to express in each swelling of the torso or the limbs the efflorescence of a muscle or a bone which lay deep beneath the skin.' Sculptor Henry Moore exercised a quite different face of spatial talent.

According to one commentator, Moore imagined the sculpture, 'whatever its size, as if he were holding it completely enclosed in the hollow of his hand; he mentally visualizes a complex form from all round itself; he knows while he looks at one side what the other side is like; he identifies himself with its center of gravity, its mass, its weight; he realizes it volume, as the space that the shape displaces in the air.'

From childhood Nikola Tesla, a mechanical engineer famous for his inventions, was tormented by sense images that were like hallucinations. 'When a word was spoken to me the image of the object it designated would present itself vividly to my vision and sometimes I was quite unable to distinguish whether what I saw was tangible or not.' To obtain some relief from these hallucinatory images, Tesla made up imaginary worlds and took make-believe journeys. He seemed to be journeying, in fact, toward madness. Then at age seventeen Tesla discovered inventing and the potentially disastrous deficit turned into a talent. He found he could visualize in perfect detail all the parts of his inventions, even testing them in his mind. He said the mental image was so real he could even note if the machine was out of balance. He claimed that if he could get an invention to run in his mind, it always ran on the workbench.

Einstein told the following story in an unpublished essay, uncovered in the Princeton archives, regarding his discovery of the general relativity theory. In the context of a specific electromagnetic problem and his struggle to understand gravity's relation to special relativity, Einstein had what he called 'the happiest thought of my life.' He suddenly *imagined* a person falling freely from the roof of a house and realized that his observer would not experience a gravitational field in his immediate vicinity. 'If the observer releases any objects,' he wrote, 'they will remain relative to him in a state of rest, or in a state of uniform motion.' That imaged thought led him to realize that gravitation and acceleration must be equivalent. His visual image provided him with the imaginal representation of simultaneous opposition."

Indeed, imagery was surely the *germ* of Einstein's discovery. The imaged gestalt— the primary focus of development in the Visualizing/Verbalizing program—is a *germ of cognition*. From it, recall, conclusion, inference, prediction, analysis, application, evaluation, and synthesis can be developed. In short, analytical thinking and comprehension can be developed.

Following the specifics in this book, the Visualizing/Verbalizing process can significantly change the life of an individual. Here are a few examples. Although not developed to a genius state, they experienced an improved quality of life and self-confidence.

Tim was a twelve-year-old, completing seventh grade, and failing his classes. His oral vocabulary was at a 15-9 mental age level, but his oral language comprehension was at an 11-6 mental age level. He spelled at a 7.9 grade level, recognized words at a high school level, had word attack skills at a 12.9 grade level, and a paragraph reading score at a 12.0 grade level. But, though he could read the high school paragraphs, his paragraph recall was unstable at the fourth grade passage.

Tim had V/V therapy in June and July, one hour a day, with good progress noted, but treatment was discontinued due to financial and time constraints. A retest at that time noted that he had improved during the two months of treatment but his imaging and language processing were not yet automatic, thus he had to reread or slow down to connect to language. I urged his family to reactivate treatment when they were able. A few months later, V/V therapy was reactivated for three months, again at one hour a day. He began to *automatically* process language. Retesting indicated that his oral language comprehension progressed to a 15-6 mental age level (previously at an 11-6 age level), he comprehended through the tenth grade passage (previously unstable at the fourth grade level), and he performed at the *98th percentile* in reading comprehension. He had remarkable interpretive comprehension skills.

And, recall the situation of Catherine from the first chapter? Interestingly enough, I recently worked with another Catherine. The parallels are uncanny, even down to the same name. Her education profile was very similar to the original Catherine, only she was in sixth grade instead of twelfth. On June 30th she was 10-8 chronologically, completing the fifth grade, and struggling in school. She was performing at a 7 year-old level in oral language comprehension (three years below her age level) and the *25th percentile* in reading comprehension (very weak). Her parents described her as having "poor retention of what she reads" and "nervous, as evidenced by nail-biting." Her year-end school testing indicated weakness in reading comprehension.

We worked with this Catherine in the V/V process one hour a day, and on October 27th, four months later, she was performing at a 14-year-old level in oral language comprehension and the *75th percentile* in reading comprehension. She demonstrated remarkable ability in comprehending language. During the post testing, she was able to answer all the comprehension questions, interpretive not just recall, on the eighth grade paragraphs. She was getting A's on social studies tests, whereas before she was barely passing. She was verbal, and her face and posture were confident and happy. I recall walking by a V/V session and she was animatedly saying to her clinician, "Come on... Aren't we going to answer those questions?" He chuckled.

And, what happened to the original Catherine? Recall that she was in twelfth grade and performing at the *9th percentile* in oral reading comprehension and the *10th percentile* in silent reading comprehension. She had only 30 minutes a day of V/V from February through May—four months with *intermittent* attendance. In May, her imaging and language processing were not yet automatic and treatment should have continued, but she decided to stop due to the onset of summer and her desire to get away from "school."

Although not finished, she improved in her ability to comprehend and connect to language. On the retest, she performed at the *37th percentile* in oral reading comprehension and the *39th percentile* in silent reading comprehension. These scores indicated moderate rather than very severe weakness. One professional described this as improvement from the "retarded" range (below the 10th percentile) to the "low normal" range (only modestly below the 50th percentile). However, though Catherine had improved, she had not stabilized, as she might have with only a few more months of treatment. She also did not graduate from high school. After twelve years of school, she wanted "out." I have often wondered what might have happened if Catherine had been worked with years earlier? Would she have responded in sixth grade like the Catherine I described on the previous page?

The individuals described above improved due to cognitive retraining from the V/V process. The most effective learning comes from experience and visualizing is a *vicarious experience*. It is not a learning style nor a learning tool. It is cognition. "It is not difficult to see why these effects are so all-inclusive when we realize that Visualizing/Verbalizing is teaching a process that is fundamental to language, not just reading," Truch (1991).

Visualizing and Verbalizing helps the brain *see*.

APPENDIX A

Summary Pages

Summary of Climate

step 1

• *Keep the climate presentation short and succinct.*

Explain *what* will do:

1. Diagram right/left hemisphere of the brain.

2. Introduce concept of right hemisphere linked to imaging.

3. Introduce concept of left hemisphere linked to talking.

4. Show how both sides work together. Introduce the phrase "Visualizing and Verbalizing" or "picturing and talking about."

Explain *why* will do it:

5. Explain that visualizing improves the ability to understand/remember what we read/hear.

6. Explain that verbalizing improves the ability to express ourselves orally or in writing.

Optional:

7. Present a reduced climate presentation for young or severely disabled students.

8. Explain that gesturing is important because it enhances oral expression.

Summary of Picture to Picture

step 2

Objective: The student will be able to give a *detailed* verbal description of a simple picture. ***Present structure words: what, size, color, number, shape, where, movement, mood, background, perspective, when, sound.***

1. The student verbally describes a simple, colored picture.

2. The teacher questions with choice and contrast to develop and refine verbalizing.

3. The student checks through the structure words, quickly reverbalizing each element.

4. The teacher summaries, using the phrase: *"Your words made me picture...."*

5. The teacher sees the picture and discusses it with the student.

6. Use simple, colored pictures with little detail and background.

7. Practice picture to picture until the student is comfortable with the task. Overlap to next step—*Word Imaging*—while continuing to practice.

8. Practice gesturing of simple objects and sentences—optional.

9. **Group Instruction:**
   Small groups of 3 to 5 are recommended. The group represents a collective individual so the interaction is similar to one-to-one. For example: Show a picture to all 5 students. Randomly choose students to describe the picture and check through structure words. This allows all students to participate and you only receive (visualize) one picture.

Summary of Word Imaging

step 3

Objective: The student will be able to visualize and verbalize, with *detail*, a single word.

1. **Object Imaging** (optional)

   a. Object imaging is for students who have difficulty understanding what it is to image.
   b. The student looks at an object, closes eyes, recalls and describes image.

2. **Personal Imaging** (not optional but only do one or two)

   a. The student recalls, images, and describes something personal but simple such as a pet, room, toy, etc.
   b. The teacher questions with choice and contrast.
   c. The structure words are checked through for details and re-verbalization.
   d. The teacher gives a verbal summary using the phrase: "Your words made me picture..."

3. **Known Noun Imaging** (*not optional*)

   a. The student visualizes and verbalizes a noun. The word should be familiar as well as high in imagery.
   b. The teacher questions specifically with choice and contrast to develop detailed imagery.
   c. The structure words are checked through for details and re-verbalization.
   d. If student has been given a choice, have the student describe the image to be sure not restating or paraphrasing.
   e. Request gesturing.
   f. Conclude session with a verbal summary using the phrase: *"Your words made me picture..."*
   g. Practice this step until very confident.

4. **Fantasy Imaging** (optional)

   a. Begin with a "known noun" image and interact to create fanciful, humorous images.
   b. Encourage student to create own fantasy images.

5. **Group Instruction:**
Apply this step to small groups of 3 to 5 students. Give one word to be described by all individuals in the group. Set the task as: *All students will help create one composite image, not separate images.* Each student will take a turn visualizing and verbalizing different aspects of the word to the group. The teacher will question, choose individuals to go through 3 or 4 structure words at a time, visualize, and summarize the composite image.

Summary of Single Sentence Imaging

step 4

Objective: The student will be able to visualize and verbalize a sentence.

1. Single sentence imaging

    a. Overlap from a *known noun* to create a simple sentence.
    b. The student images parts of a sentence—words—to construct a sentence gestalt.
    c. Include *detailed imagery*.
    d. Include fanciful images by constructing a simple + silly sentence.

2. Underlining image words

    a. Student underlines the image words while reading the sentence orally.
    b. Do not teach a grammar lesson.

Note: The single sentence imaging step is optional. This type of stimulation often only requires modest attention or may be omitted completely.

Summary of Sentence by Sentence Imaging

step 5

Objective: The student will image a paragraph gestalt by visualizing and verbalizing each sentence of a paragraph, then verbalizing a picture summary and word summary.

1. The student images each sentence to create a paragraph gestalt.

2. The teacher interacts by questioning to develop an imaged gestalt.

3. The structure words are checked through for the first sentence to develop detailed imagery for topic sentence.

4. The student gives a *picture summary*—touches each felt and says: "Here I saw... "

5. The student gives a *word summary*—a verbal summary that uses images to formulate generalizations.

6. The sentence images build on one another rather than separate parts.

7. Question or comment with choice and contrast to create images for the student. Follow each sentence stimulus with: "What do those words make you picture?"

8. Be alert to paraphrasing, rather than imaging.

9. Begin receptively—you read each sentence to the student. Later the student will read each sentence orally or silently, continuing the same general technique of giving a picture and word summary.

10. Begin to diagnose for automatic imaging.

11. Initially, use low-level material, despite age or grade level. Increase the paragraph difficulty as the student acquires proficiency.

12. Present material in all three modes:
    a. You read each sentence to the student (receptive)
    b. Student reads each sentence aloud (expressive)

      c. Student reads each sentence to self (same procedure of placing colored square and verbalizing images)

13. Correct picture summaries by cuing the student with a part of the image.

14. Correct word summaries by using the phrase: "Your words made me picture..." Spice up an erroneous image to encourage the student to be specific with the verbalization.

15. Reread a sentence to clarify a specific image.

16. *Sentence by sentence level is critical—practice vigorously.*

17. **Group Instruction:**
Consider the small group—3 to 5 students—a collective individual. All students participate in the same paragraph. Choose a different student to: 1) visualize and verbalize each sentence, 2) check through the structure words on first sentence, 3) verbalize the picture summary, and 4) verbalize the word summary.

Summary of Sentence by Sentence with HOTS

step 6

Objective: The student will be able to visualize and verbalize sentence-by-sentence, continuing to develop a paragraph gestalt, and *begin* to develop higher order thinking skills.

1. The student visualizes each sentence to create a paragraph gestalt, using colored squares.

2. The teacher interacts, *beginning* to ask open-ended questions rather than choice/contrast questions.

3. The structure words might be used for first sentence.

4. The student verbalizes a *picture summary*.

5. The student verbalizes a *word summary*.

6. The student verbalizes the *main idea* from the imaged gestalt.

   a. Stimulate main idea generalizing with the principle of contrast and choice.
   b. Stimulate main idea generalizing by initiating a part of it.

7. The teacher asks "why" questions to stimulate an *inference* from the imaged gestalt.

8. The teacher asks questions from the imaged gestalt that will stimulate the student's ability to *draw conclusions and predict/extend* information.

9. Consider the issue of *lesson energy*.

10. Remember to diagnose for automatic imaging *as* language is received.

11. Remember to require the student to receive language in all three modes: receptive—aloud—to self.

12. **Group Instruction:**
    Consider the small group—3 to 5 students—a collective individual. All students participate in the same paragraph. Choose a different student to 1) visualize and verbalize each sentence, 2) check through structure words on

first sentence, 3) verbalize picture summary and word summary, and 4) respond to interpretive questions.

Summary of Multiple Sentence Imaging

step 7

Objective: The student will be able to visualize and verbalize, *with automaticity,* from two or more sentences at a time, verbalizing word summaries and answering higher order thinking skill questions.

1. This step is a modified format of sentence by sentence imaging.

2. The goal is to continue constructing imaged gestalts from larger and larger "parts."

3. The student receives or reads two sentences, a third, or half the paragraph.

4. *The structure words are obsolete.*

5. The use of the colored squares is recommended.

6. Include a picture summary.

7. Include a word summary to generalize the imaged gestalt.

8. The student will visualize and verbalize more easily now and require less questioning and stimulation.

9. Note whether the student is visualizing and verbalizing with automaticity *as* the language enters his or her mind.

10. Ask interpretive comprehension questions of *main idea, inference, conclusion, prediction.*

11. Use all three modes of receiving language: receptive, aloud, self.

12. **Group Instruction:**
    Choose a different student to 1) V/V each part of the paragraph, 2) give the picture summary, 3) give the word summary, and 4) answer interpretive questions.

Summary of Whole Paragraph Imaging

step 8

Objective: The student will be able to visualize and verbalize a whole paragraph with automaticity, refined verbal summaries, and good interpretive higher order comprehension.

1. This step modifies the format of previous levels, thus is easily mastered by all.

2. The student reads and/or receives a whole paragraph of content.

3. *No colored squares or structure words are necessary.*

4. *No picture summary.* Instead, the student describes specific images *after* giving a word summary.

5. The student verbalizes a *refined* word summary.

6. **Ask interpretive comprehension questions to be answered from the imaged gestalt.**

    * **Main idea**
    * **Inference**
    * **Conclusion**
    * **Predict/extend**
    * **Evaluate**

7. Diagnose whether the student is imaging automatically. Note gesturing, eye movement, or response to content as the individual receives language.

8. Use all three modes of receiving language:

    * receptive—you read to the student
    * expressive—student reads aloud
    * expressive— student reads to self

9. The student may reread all or part of the content in order to image.

10. Although imaging is more automatic and assumed at this level, question specifics to determine that the individual is actually imaging and not just restating sentences or paraphrasing.

11. **Group Instruction:**
One student reads or receives the entire paragraph and gives a word summary. Teacher and other students question for imaging. Students take turns responding to interpretive questions.

Summary of Paragraph by Paragraph Imaging

step 9

Objective: The student will be able to visualize and verbalize a whole page of written material (one paragraph at a time), give a general page summary, and answer interpretive, higher order comprehension questions.

1. The student receives or reads entire paragraph.

2. The student verbalizes a word summary per paragraph, placing a colored square.

3. The teacher checks for specific images, but primarily assumes imaging.

4. The student touches each colored square and gives a *page summary* of the entire page of material.

5. The student reads aloud or silently, with the emphasis on the latter. Include receptive stimulation to continue aiding the student in processing oral language.

6. *It is imperative to continue interpretive questions of main idea, inference, conclusion, prediction, and evaluation.*

7. Group Instruction:
   Each student reads or receives one paragraph, places a colored square, and gives paragraph word summary. Choose one student to give a page summary and different students to answer interpretive questions.

Summary of Whole Page Imaging

step 10

Objective: The student will be able to visualize and verbalize a page of written material, give a *refined* page summary, and answer oral and written interpretive comprehension questions.

1. V/V continues with larger and larger units of language—a whole page.

2. Detailed imagery is not necessary unless there is some question as to whether the student is not imaging automatically.

3. The student verbalizes a *refined* page summary.

4. The student is moved into higher grade levels as well as denser and different types of material. Extend to content areas.

5. The primary focus is on silent reading, but pursue some receptive stimulation to continue stimulating oral language comprehension and prepare for note taking lectures.

6. The student is now *automatically* interpreting the content, preferably without prompting or questioning. ***The goal is to refine verbalization and higher order thinking skills.***

Summary of Chapter and Lecture Noting

step 11

Objective: The student will apply V/V to noting oral and written material by analyzing and capturing critical concepts for further study or memorization.

1. Notes reduce content to a size that can be learned, memorized, and retrieved.

2. Explain the need for chapter noting:

   a. Read a chapter only once for an exam.
   b. Reduce numerous pages of content to only a few pages.

3. Scan the chapter for preparatory images.

4. Teach a modified outline technique:

   a. Use general outline of headings or lists.
   b. Indent details.
   c. Enlarge specifics.
   d. List information to be memorized.
   e. Use equal sign or colon.w

5. Model and practice the noting procedure for written language.

   a. Student verbalizes what to include, you write the notes.
   b. You verbalize what to include, student writes the notes.
   c. You and student each read and write notes, comparing which would be easier to study.
   d. Student reads and notes, you give feedback.

6. Extend to practicing noting oral language.

   a. Explore difference between noting oral and written language.
   b. Explore need for brevity in note taking, questioning for example, and need to create imaginal representations.
   c. Deformalize written language for lecturing, begin with one page and extend to mock lectures of 5 to 10 minutes.
   d. Review students' notes, interact, recognize areas of strength and weakness.
   e. Practice, practice, practice....

Summary of Writing from Visualizing/Verbalizing

step 12

1. Stimulate gestalt processing.
   Develop thinking and oral language comprehension and oral language expression by using the Visualizing/Verbalizing program. This will develop a language base from which writing can be taught.

2. Begin teaching the "parts" for writing.
   Teach sentence structure, basic punctuation, and spelling.

3. Teach paragraph Writing.
   While teaching sentence structure, punctuation, and spelling, overlap to the following:

   a. Paragraph copying.

   b. Paragraph editing—specify if editing for spelling, sentence structure, punctuation, organization, or all of the preceding.

   c. Paragraph summary from V/V image-cue cards. Write and edit.

   d. Paragraph summary without cue cards. Write and edit.

   e. Paragraph summary from scratch—use free writing and clustering.

   f. Page summary with image-cue cards. Write and edit.

   g. Expository paragraphs using specific format for organization and focus. Write and edit.

   h. Narrative paragraphs using specific format for organization and focus. Write and edit.

APPENDIX B

Picture to Picture Illustrations

This section has illustrations adapted from the
Romney Gay Alphabet Book
and
original drawings by Phyllis Lindamood.

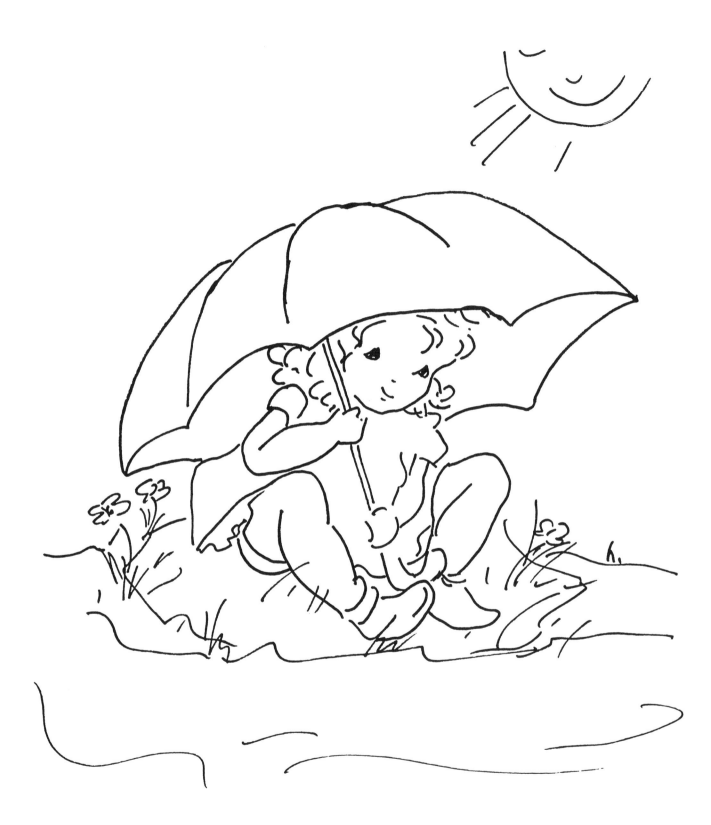

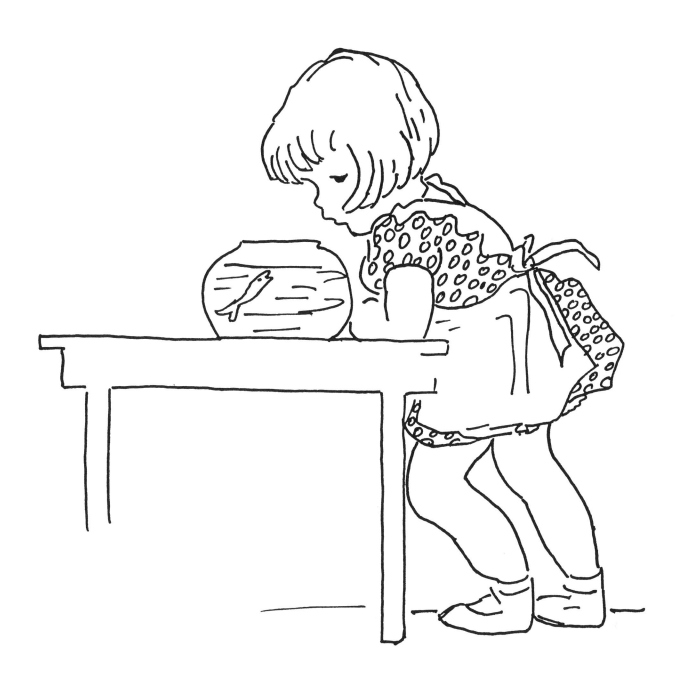

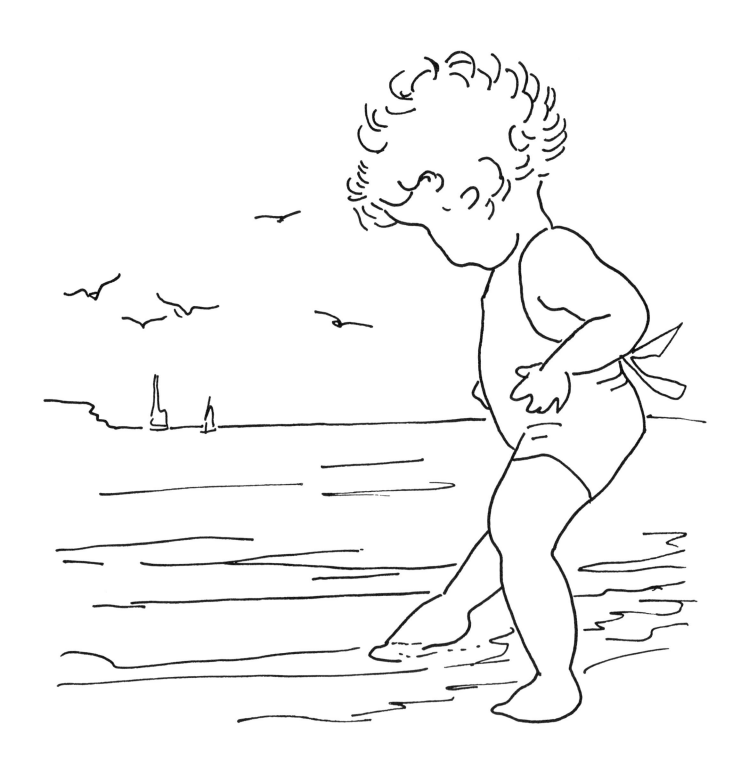

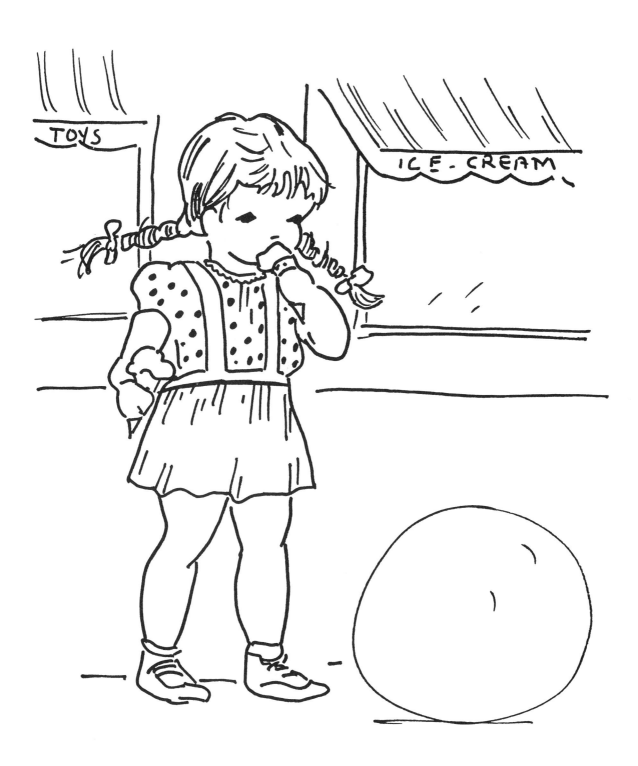

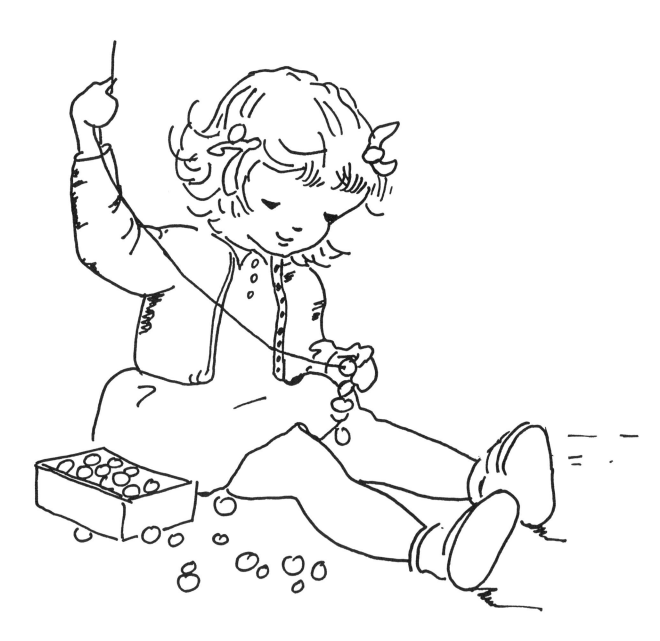

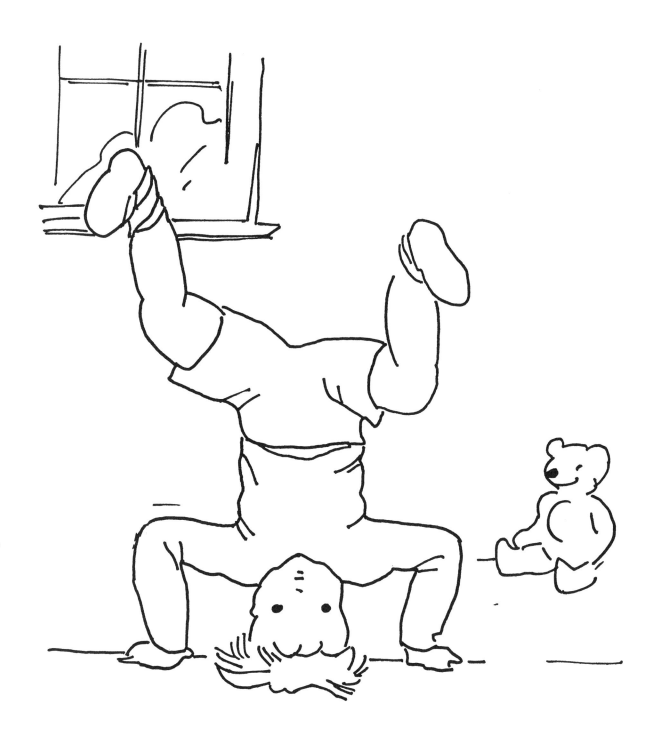

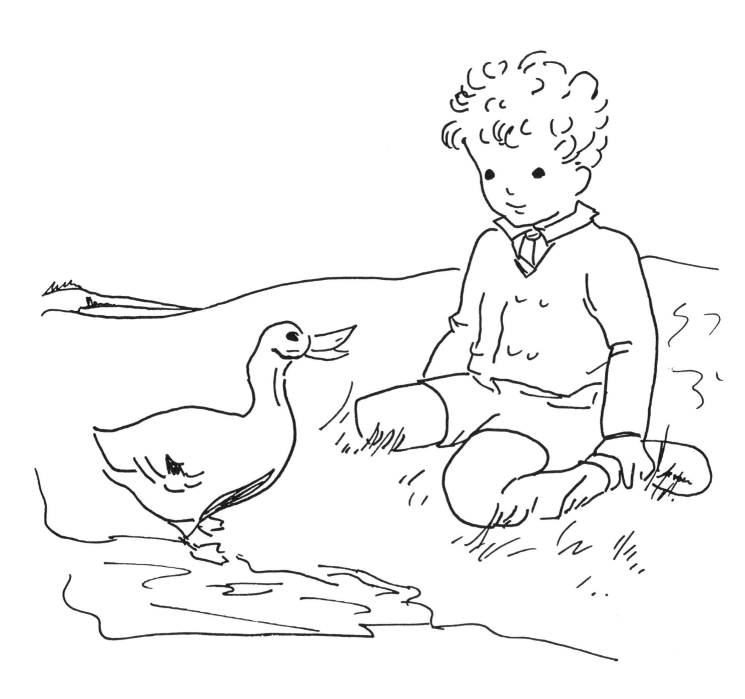

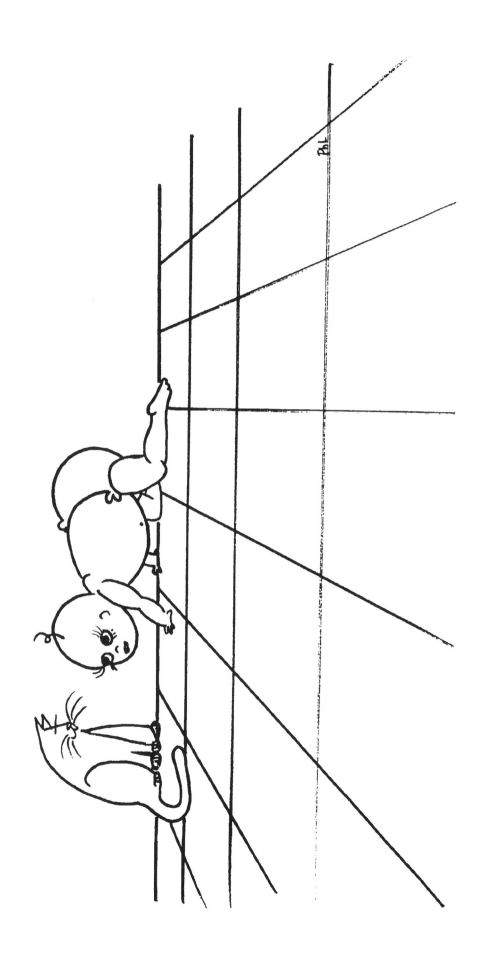

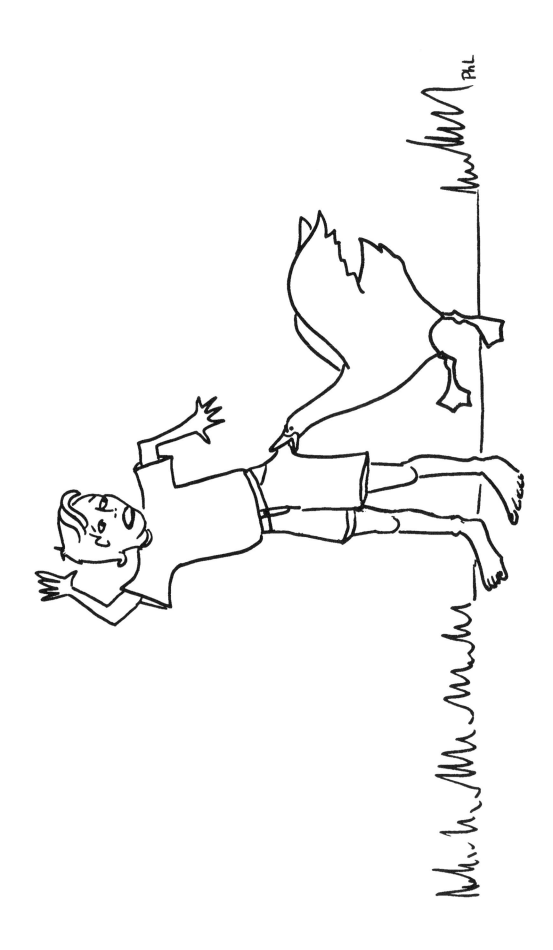

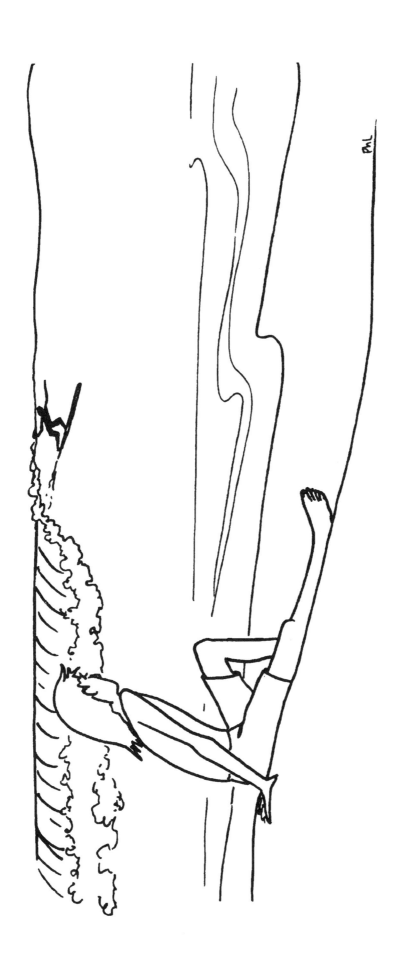

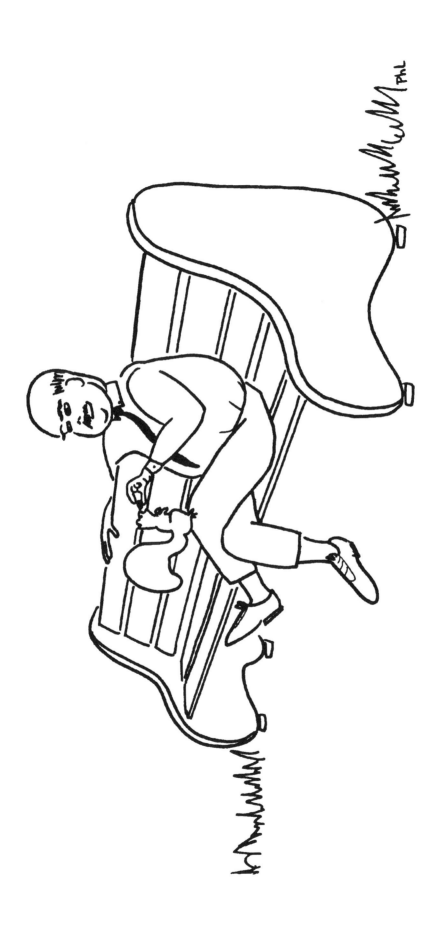

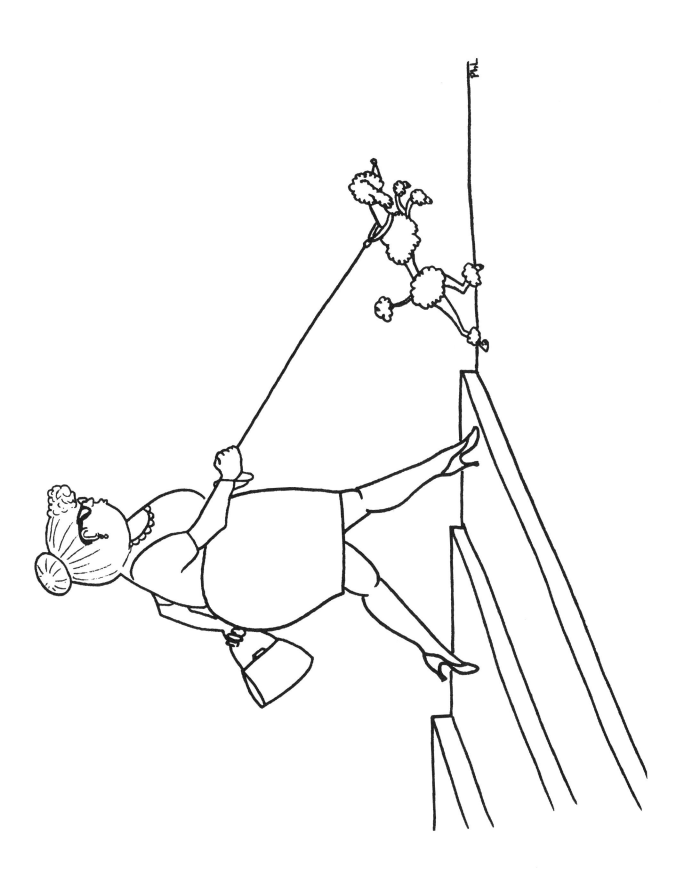

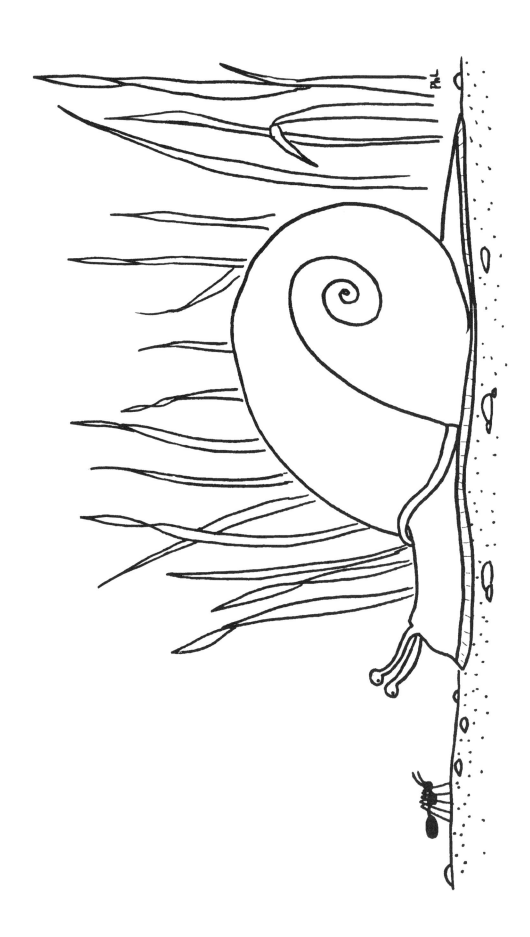

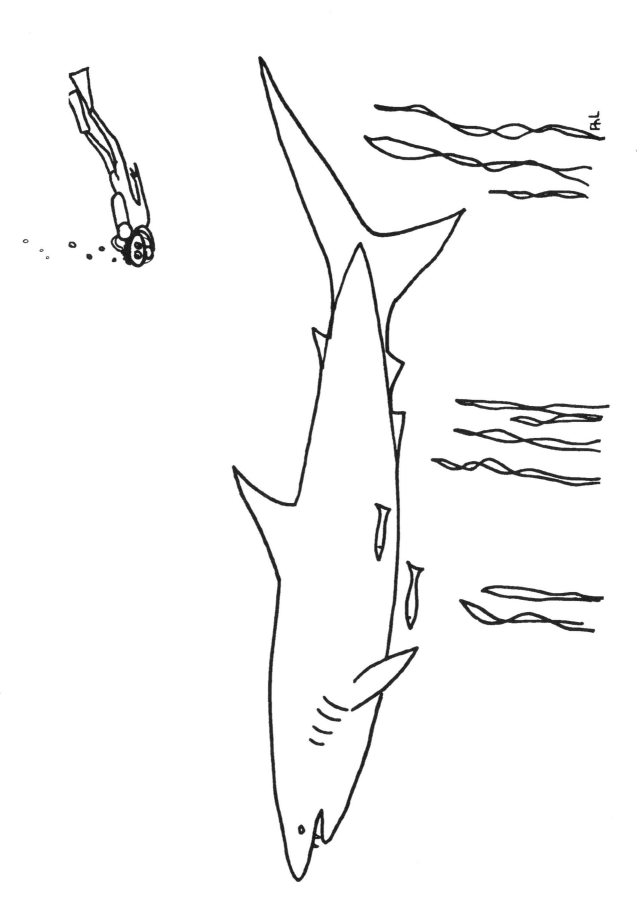

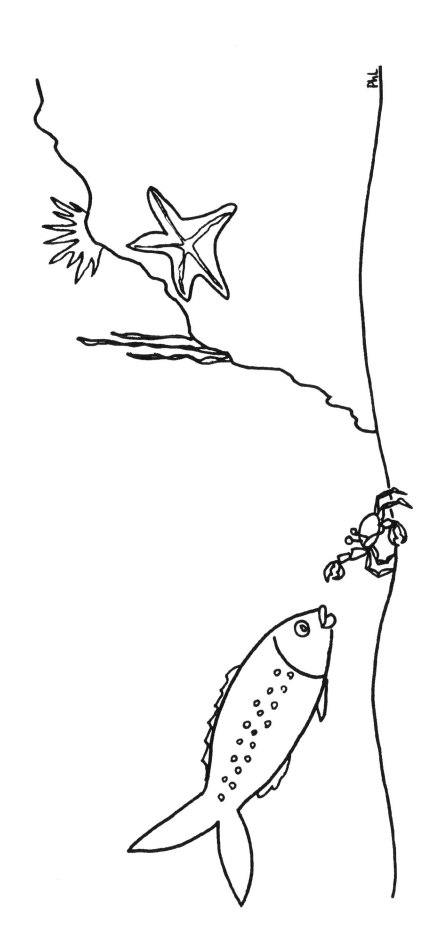

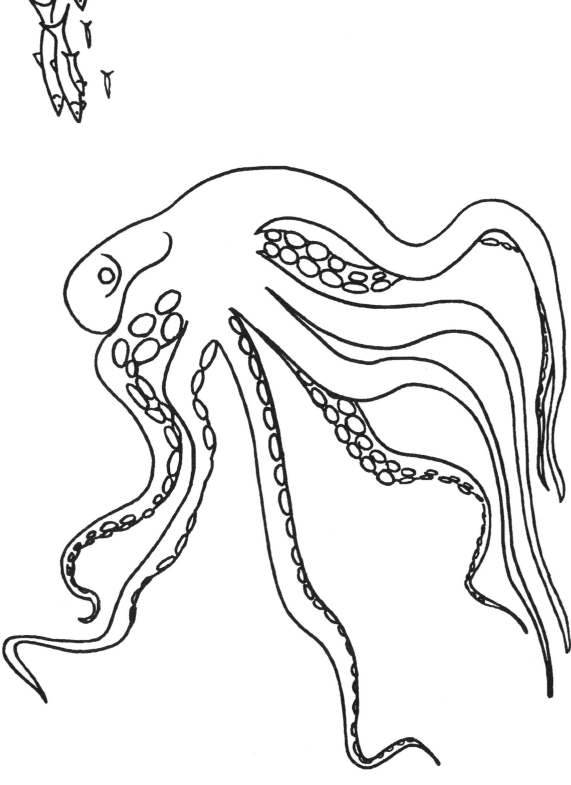

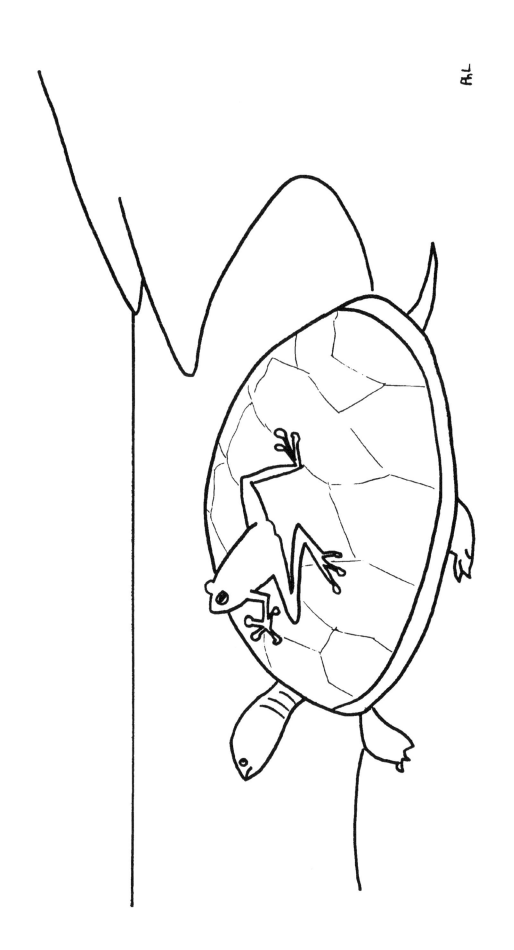

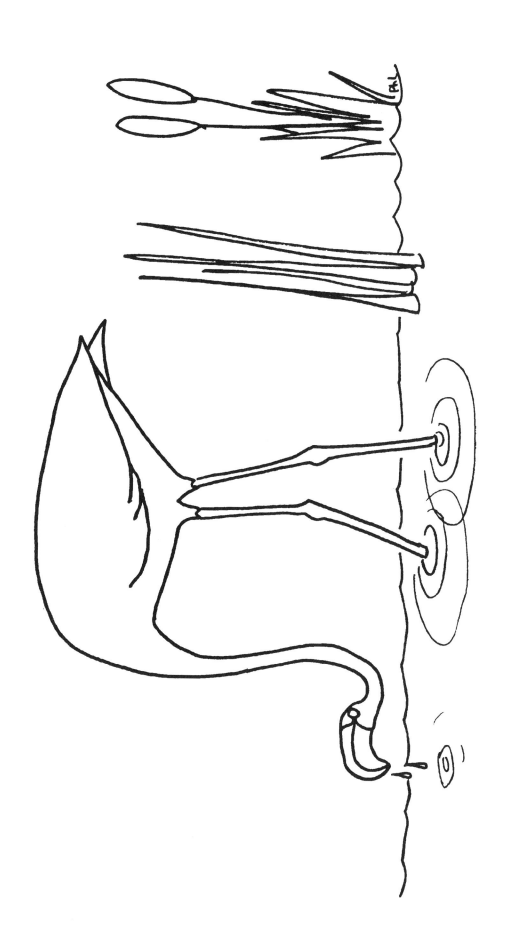

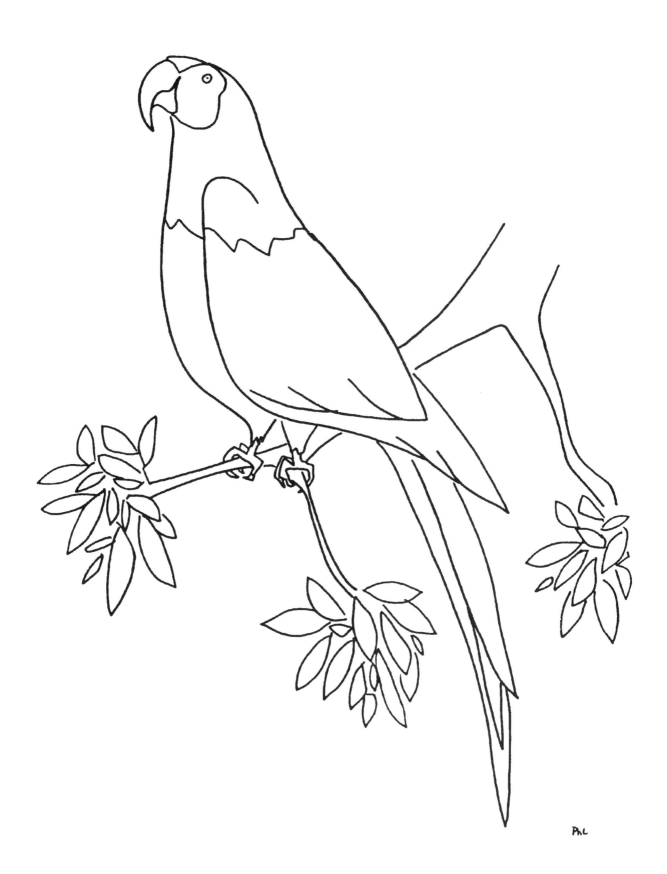

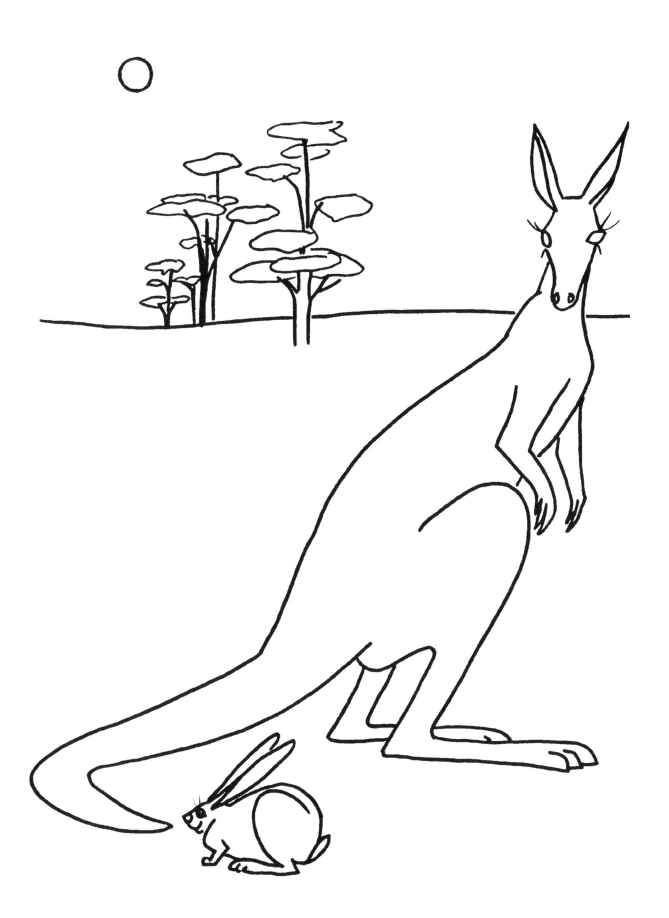

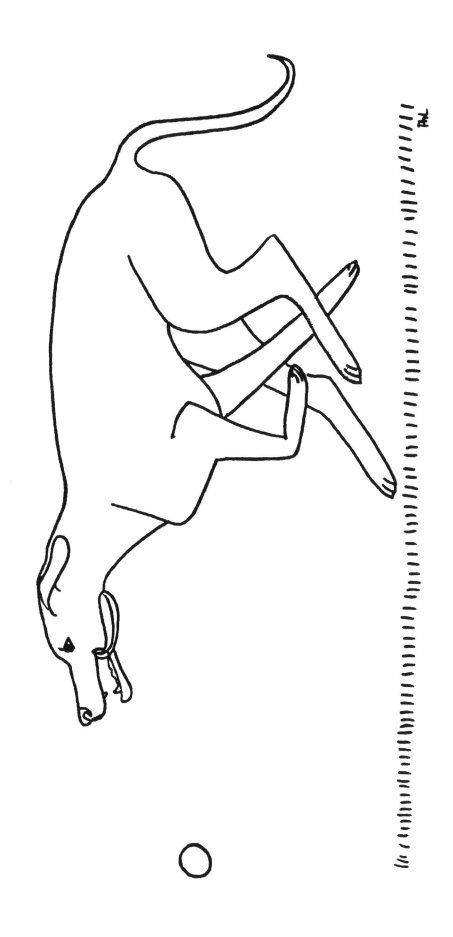

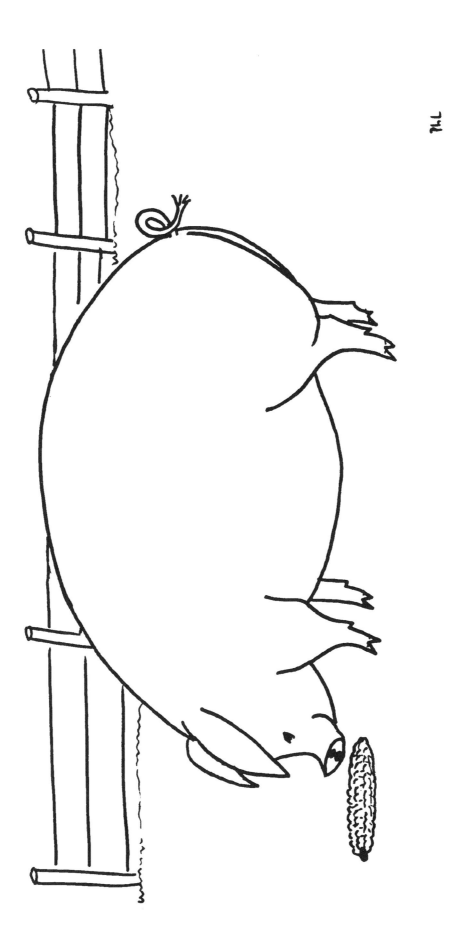

V/V Checklist and Structure Words

1 what	7 movement
2 size	8 mood
3 color	9 background
4 number	10 perspective
5 shape	11 when
6 where	12 sound

Visualizing/Verbalizing Checklist

Picture to Picture
1. Structure words used = ☐some ☐all
2. Questioning needed = ☐lots ☐some ☐none
3. Verbalizing = ☐poor ☐ok ☐fluent

Word Imaging
1. Structure words used = ☐some ☐all
2. Questioning needed = ☐lots ☐some
3. Imagery = ☐weak ☐ok ☐detailed

Sentence x Sentence — Multiple Sentence

Level		D	G	PS	WS	MI	I	DC	R & E
C	S x S / MS x MS								
D	S x S / MS x MS								
E	S x S / MS x MS								
F	S x S / MS x MS								
G	S x S / MS x MS								
H	S x S / MS x MS								
I	S x S / MS x MS								
J	S x S / MS x MS								
K	S x S / MS x MS								
L	S x S / MS x MS								

Legend:
- D = details
- G = gestalt
- PS = picture summary
- WS = word summary
- MI = main idea
- I = inference
- DC = draw conclusion
- R & E = receptive expressive

Whole Paragraph — Paragraph x Paragraph

Level		G	FWS	✔Image	MI	I	DC	R & E
C	¶ / ¶ x ¶							
D	¶ / ¶ x ¶							
E	¶ / ¶ x ¶							
F	¶ / ¶ x ¶							
G	¶ / ¶ x ¶							
H	¶ / ¶ x ¶							
I	¶ / ¶ x ¶							
J	¶ / ¶ x ¶							
K	¶ / ¶ x ¶							
L	¶ / ¶ x ¶							

Legend:
FWS = fluent word summary

Aristotle. <u>Aristotle on Memory.</u> Providence, Rhode Island: Brown University Press, 1972.

Arnheim, Rudolph. "Image and Thought." <u>In</u> G. Kepes (ed.). <u>Sign, Image, Symbol,</u> New York: George Braziller, Inc., 1966.

Arnheim, Rudolf. <u>Visual Thinking</u>. Los Angeles, California: University of California Press, 1969.

Bell, Nanci. "Gestalt Imagery: A Critical Factor in Language Comprehension." <u>In</u> Press. <u>Annals of Dyslexia,</u> Baltimore, M.D. : Orton Dyslexia Society, 1991.

Bleasdale, F. "Paivio's Dual-Coding Model of Meaning Revisited." <u>In</u> J. C. Yuille (ed.). <u>Imagery, Memory and Cognition: Essays in honor of Allan Paivio,</u> New Jersey: Lawrence Erlbaum Associates, 1978.

Boning, Richard. <u>Specific Skills Series.</u> New York: Barnell Loft, Ltd., 1970.

Boning, Richard. <u>Multiple Skills Series</u>. New York: Barnell Loft, Ltd., 1977.

Bosshardt, H.G. "The Influence of Visual and Auditory Images on Visual and Auditory Word Identification." <u>Psychological Research,</u> 1975.

Bower, Gordon H., and D.G. Morrow. "Mental Models in Narrative Comprehension." <u>Science,</u> (January 1990) : 44-48.

Briggs, John. <u>Fire in the Crucible, The Alchemy of Creative Genius.</u> New York: St. Martin's Press, 1988.

Britcher, Phyllis. <u>The Romney Gay ABC</u>. New York: Grosset and Dunlap, 1946.

Burns, Edward. <u>Western Civilization</u>. New York: W.W. Norton & Company, Inc.,1958.

Buzan, Tony. <u>Use Both Sides of Your Brain</u>. New York: E.D. Burton, New York, 1976.

Changeux, Jean-Pierre. <u>Neuronal Man: The Biology of Mind</u>. New York: Pantheon Books, 1985.

Clark, James M., and Allan Paivio. "Dual Coding Theory and Education." <u>In</u> press, <u>Educational Psychology Review,</u> September 1991.

Fokes, Joann. Fokes Sentence Builder. DLM Allen, Texas: Teaching Resources,1976.

Foley, M. A., and A. Wilder.   "Developmental Comparisons of the Effects of Type of Imaginal Elaboration on Memory." Paper read at the Biennial Meeting of the Society for Research in Child Development, April 1989, Kansas City, Mo.

Fry, Edward.   Reading Drills for Speed and Comprehension. Providence, Rhode Island: Jamestown Publishers, 1975.

Fry, Edward.   Vocabulary Drills. Providence, Rhode Island: Jamestown Publishers, 1986.

Geschwind, Norman.   Selected Papers on Language and the Brain. Boston, Mass.: D. Reidel Publishing, 1974.

Glazier, Teresa   The Least You Should Know about English. New York: CBS College Publishing, Holt, Rinehart, and Winston, 1979.

Healy, Jane M.   Endangered Minds: Why Our Children Don't Think. New York: Simon and Schuster, 1990.

Hechinger, F.   "About education." New York Times, March 16, 1988.

Horgan, John.   "Profile: Physicist John A. Wheeler." Scientific American, June, 1991.

Katz, Albert N., and Allan Paivio.   "Imagery Variables in Concept Identification." Journal of Verbal Learning and Verbal Behavior, June 1975.

Kimbrough, Judy.   Interview with Paul E. Worthington, Window Rock Elementary School, Window Rock, Arizona, 1991.

Konicek, Richard D.   "Seeking Synergism for Man's Two-hemisphere Brain." Phi Delta Kappan, September 1975.

Kosslyn, Stephen M.   "Information Representation in Visual Images." Cognitive Psychology, July 1975.

Kosslyn, Stephen M.   "Using Imagery to Retrieve Semantic Information: A Developmental Study." Child Development, June 1976.

Kosslyn, Stephen M.   Ghosts in the Minds Machine. New York: W.W. Norton, 1983.

Kosslyn, Stephen M.   "Stalking the Mental Image." Psychology Today, May 1985.

Laughlin, Charles D., John McManus, Eugene G. d'Aquili.   Brain, Symbol and Experience. Boston, Mass: Shambhala Publications, Inc.,1990.

Levin, J.R.   "Inducing Comprehension in Poor Readers." Journal of Educational Psychology, 65 (1973): 19-24.

Levin, J.R.   "On Functions of Pictures in Prose." In F. Pirozzolo & M. Wittrock (eds.). Neuropsychological and Cognitive Processes in Reading, New York: Academic Press, 1981.

Levy, Jerre.   "Right Brain Left Brain: Fact and Fiction." Psychology Today, May 1985.

Lindamood, Charles and Patricia.   Auditory Discrimination in Depth. Allen,Texas: DLM Teaching Resources, 1969.

Linden, M.A. and Merlin Wittrock.   "The Teaching of Reading Comprehension According to the Model of Generative Learning". Reading Research Quarterly, 17 (1981): 44-57.

Long, S.A., P.N. Winograd, and C.A. Bridge.   "The Effects of Reader and Text Characteristics on Reports of Imagery During and After Reading." Reading Research Quarterly,19(1989): 353-372.

Macht, Michael., and James C. Scheirer.   "The Effect of Imagery on Accessability and Availability in a Short-term Memory Paradigm." Verbal Learning and Verbal Behavior, October 1975.

Marks, D.F.   "Vividness of Visual Imagery and Effect on Function." In P. Sheehan (ed.). The Function and Nature of Imagery, New York: Academic Press, 1972.

Morris, P.E., and P. J. Hampson.   Imagery and Consciousness. New York: Academic Press, 1983.

Oliver, M.E.   "Improving Comprehension with Mental Imagery." Paper read at the Annual Meeting of the Washington Organization for Reading Development of the International Reading Association, Seattle, Washington, March 1982.

Ornstein, Robert.   "The Split and the Whole Brain." Human Nature, May 1978.

Paivio, Allan.   "Mental Imagery in Associative Learning and Memory." Psychological Review, 76 (1969): 241-263.

Paivio, Allan. <u>Imagery and Verbal Processes.</u> New York: Holt, Rinehart, and Winston, 1971. Reprinted, Hillsdale New Jersey: Lawrence Erlbaum Associates, 1979.

Paivio, Allan. <u>Mental Representations: A Dual Coding Approach</u>. New York: Oxford University Press, 1986.

Parks, A. Franklin, Jame Levernier, and Ida Hollowell. <u>Structuring Paragraphs</u>. New York: St. Martin's Press, 1981.

Pauk, Walter. <u>Six-Way Paragraphs</u>. Providence, Rhode Island: Jamestown Publishers, 1983.

Peters, E.E., and J. R. Levin. "Effects of a Mnemonic Imagery Strategy on Good and Poor Readers' Prose Recall." <u>Reading Research Quarterly</u>, 21 (1986):179-192.

Piaget, Jean., and Inhelder Barbel. <u>The Psychology of the Child</u>. New York: Basic Books, Inc., 1969.

Piaget, Jean and B. Inhelder. <u>Imagery and the Child</u>. New York: Basic Books, Inc., 1971.

Pietsch, Paul. "The Optics of Memory." <u>Wraparound, Harpers</u>, Dec. 1975.

Pirozzolo, F. and Merlin Wittrock. <u>Neuropsychological and Cognitive Processes in Reading</u>. New York: Academic Press, Inc., 1981.

Pressley, G.M. "Mental Imagery Helps Eight-year Olds Remember What They Read." <u>Journal of Educational Psychology,</u> 68 (1976): 355-359.

Pribram, Karl. <u>Languages of the Brain: Experimental Paradoxes and Principles in Neuropsychology</u>. New York: Brandon House, Inc., 1971.

Richardson, A. <u>Mental Imagery</u>. London: Routledge & Kegan Paul, 1969.

Rollins, M. <u>Mental Imagery: On the Limits of Cognitive Science</u>. New Haven, Connecticut: Yale University Press, 1989.

Sadoski, Mark. "An Exploratory Study of the Relationship Between Reported Imagery and the Comprehension and Recall of a Story." <u>Reading Research Quarterly</u>, 19-1 (1983): 110-123.

Sadoski, Mark. "The Natural Use of Imagery in Story Comprehension and Recall: Replication and Extension." Reading Research Quarterly, Fall 1985.

Sadoski, Mark, Ernest T. Goetz , and Suzanne Kangiser. "Imagination in Story Response: Relationships Between Imagery, Affect, and Structural Importance." Reading Research Quarterly, Summer 1988.

Sadoski, Mark, and Zeba Quast. "Reading Response and Long-term Recall for Journalistic Text: The roles of Imagery, Affect, and Importance." Reading Research Quarterly, Fall, 1990.

Sadoski, Mark, Ernest T. Goetz, Arturo Olivarez, Sharon Lee, and Nancy M. Roberts. "Imagination in Story Reading: The Role of Imagery, Verbal Recall, Story Analysis, and Processing Levels." Journal of Reading Behavior, 1990.

Sadoski, Mark. "Text Structure, Imagery, and Affect in the Recall of a Story by children." Changing Perspective in Research in Reading/Language Processing and Instruction Thirty-third Yearbook of the National Reading Conference. Washington, D.C.: National Reading Conference.

Samples, Robert E. "Are You Teaching Only One Side of the Brain?" Learning, February 1975.

Samples, Robert E. "Learning with the Whole Brain." Human Behavior, February 1975.

Samuels, Mike and Nancy. Seeing with the Mind's Eye. New York: Random House, 1975.

Sheehan, P.W. (ed.). The Function and Nature of Imagery. New York: Academic Press, 1972.

Simon, H.A. "What is visual imagery? An information processing interpretation." In L.W. Gregg (ed.). Cognition in Learning and Memory. New York: John Wiley & Sons, Inc., 1972.

Smith, B.D., N. Stahl, and J. Neil. "The Effect of Imagery Instruction on Vocabulary Development." Journal of College Reading and Learning, 20 (1987):131-137.

Stemmler, A. "Reading of Highly Creative Versus Highly Intelligent Secondary Students." Reading and Realism, 13 (1969): 821-831.

Tierney, R.J., and J. W. Cunningham. "Research on Teaching Reading Comprehension." In P.D. Pearson (ed.). Handbook of Reading Research, New York: Longman, 1984.

Trelease, Jim. The Read Aloud Handbook. New York: Penguin Books, 1982.

Truch, Stephen. The Missing Parts of Whole Language. Calgary, Alberta Canada: Foothills Educational Materials,1991.

Untermeyer, Louis. The Golden Treasury of Poetry. New York: Golden Press, 1959.

Venezky, R., et al. The Subtle Danger. Center for the Assessment of Educational Progress, Educational Testing Service, 1987.

Wepman, Joseph M. "Aphasia: Language Without Thought or Thought Without Language?" ASHA, March 1976.

Wheatley, Grayson H., and Robert H. Frankland. "Hemispheric Specialization and Cognitive Development." Purdue University manuscript,1976.

Wicker, Frank W. "Our Picture of Mental Imagery: Prospects for Research and Development." Educational Communication and Technology, Spring 1978.

Winson, Jonathan. Brain and Psyche. New York: Anchor Press/Doubleday, 1985.

Wittrock, Merlin C. (ed.). Learning and Instruction: Readings in Educational Research. Berkeley, California: McCutcham Publishing Corp., 1977.

Wittrock, Merlin C. The Brain and Psychology. New York: Academic Press, 1980.

Wittrock, Merlin C. "The Generative Processes of Memory." Manuscript from Education Department at University of California, Los Angeles.

Workshop

Nanci Bell offers one day Nancibell™ Visualizing/Verbalizing Workshops.

The concept is presented and specific steps are practiced. The workshops are available worldwide. Call 800-233-1819 for information.

Notes—